MW01027795

# Advanced Praise for
## *Secrets of a Kosher Girl*

"*Secrets of a Kosher Girl* brings the kosher diet into modern-day practice by using its guidelines, food choices, and eating behaviors to mold it into a successful health plan."

—RABBI SHMULEY BOTEACH, author of *Kosher Sex*

"Beth Warren has been changing people's lives for nearly a decade through her nutrition practice, *Secrets of a Kosher Girl* will surely change your life, as well. It offers step-by-step recipes and enlightened tips to keep you on the path towards a healthy and balanced life."

—JAMIE GELLER, best-selling author and founder of Kosher Network International, publisher of Jamiegeller.com and FreshFamilies.us

"Along with their efforts to probe for our place and purpose, religions confer rhythms, rituals, and rules for living. Dietary rituals and rules often derive from insights about health, and lend the benefit of discipline. In this welcome and thoughtful book, Beth Warren combines the time-honored value of Kosher dietary discipline with a keen understanding of modern nutrition to craft a unique and empowering recipe."

—DR. DAVID KATZ, founder of the True Health Initiative and author of *The Truth About Food* (HarperOne; due 2018)

"Beth has taught me so much about mindful eating and taking care of myself through good dietary habits. Her second book has taken healthy eating to the next level with passion and excitement. Beth knows food and in this book she shares her approach with her readers in a fun and engaging manner."

—NAOMI NACHMAN, author of *Perfect for Pesach*

# SECRETS

*of a*

## KOSHER GIRL

# SECRETS

## *of a*

# KOSHER GIRL

### A 21-DAY NOURISHING PLAN
### TO LOSE WEIGHT AND FEEL GREAT
### *(EVEN IF YOU'RE NOT JEWISH)*

## BETH WARREN, MS, RDN, CDN

*Foreword by*
DR. JOEL KAHN, MD

A POST HILL PRESS BOOK

Secrets of a Kosher Girl:
A 21-Day Nourishing Plan to Lose Weight and Feel Great (Even If You're Not Jewish)
© 2018 by Beth Warren
All Rights Reserved

ISBN: 978-1-68261-499-0
ISBN (eBook): 978-1-68261-500-3

Cover art by Tricia Principe, principedesign.com
Photography by Moshe Wulliger
Interior design and composition by Greg Johnson, Textbook Perfect
Emojis by Freepik.com

No part of this book may be reproduced, stored in a retrieval system, or transmitted by any means without the written permission of the author and publisher.

This book contains advice and information relating to health care. It should be used to supplement rather than replace the advice of your doctor or another trained health professional. If you know or suspect that you have a health problem, it is recommended that you seek your physician's advice before embarking on any medical program or treatment. All efforts have been made to assure the accuracy of the information in this book as of the date of publication. The publisher and the author disclaim liability for any medical outcomes that may occur as a result of applying the methods suggested in this book.

**Post Hill Press**
New York • Nashville
posthillpress.com
Published in the United States of America

# Contents

# ACKNOWLEDGMENTS

The saying, "It takes a village," couldn't be more apropos when it comes to getting *Secrets of a Kosher Girl* publishing ready.

To all the dieters back when it was called "The Kosher Cleanse," and my recipe testers, nutrition and medical facts checkers, especially my team at Beth Warren Nutrition, and our hard-working interns, thank you is an understatement for the amount of support you gave me.

Thank you to the volunteers willing to look over the pages of my book, and my brother and brothers-in-law for their expertise in the world of the Talmud and Jewish thought, for without their help, this book wouldn't have as much impact. To my food photography squad, Moishe Wulliger and Renee Muller, thank you for understanding my vision and making it come to light through the incredible photos and styling.

I would also be remiss not to give an exclusive mention to my assistant, Sarah Kassin, who keeps me on my game and acts as a chameleon in the company doing whatever is needed. Her (and her Harari family) stamp is all over these recipes. Your willingness to stand by me both in our personal and professional journeys in life is something I cherish.

As for my agent, Linda Konner, your encouragement, support, and guidance helped make *Secrets of a Kosher Girl* come to fruition. Without you, there would be no "Kosher Girl," for which I am forever grateful.

To the publishing team at Post Hill Press, especially my editor, Debra Englander, thank you for believing in the concept and strategy of the kosher girl's diet. You are the reason we can spread the message and promote positive, sustainable, and healthy changes, the kosher whole foods way, to the masses. It's a dream come true.

Most importantly, to my family, the loves of my life: you are my pillars of strength. I feel so lucky to have such incredible support from you to do what I do both inside and outside the home. My dear kids, Rivkah,

Channah, Aryeh, Levana, and Noa, thank you for your happy smiles, funny laughs, and even your tears shed on our experiences together, especially taste testing Mommy's recipes and the help you give cooking and baking too. You forever will make me proud to do the best job I have...be a mommy to you.

Finally, thanks to the number one man supporting me in everything I do, my husband, Elliot. Your partnership with me in my personal and professional life is what drives me to pursue my goals. You kept me motivated and inspired by being you, plus your encouragement of this book and belief in my career helps solidify my aspirations in helping people through the power of food.

# The Essence of Kosher and Health

Dr. Joel Kahn, MD

The miracle of the human body is easy to overlook. The fact that trillions of cells are working 24/7 to break down molecules from our food, our air, and our skin is truly an amazing thought. Thousands of enzymes are working to transform these chemicals into nourishing products to enrich our health or to worsen it. Silently, we are a chemistry lab every day.

I have been fascinated by this during my many-decade career as a preventive cardiologist and university professor. A mindfulness of these processes leads to a thought: does the quality of our food, our air, and chemicals contacting our skin matter for health? Indeed, in the last twenty years, we have come to understand that we can control so much of our health by appreciating that what we let into our body can make a huge impact on how we feel and the actual number of years we have to feel that way.

I grew up in a kosher home and continue to observe kosher dietary laws more than six decades later. I am grateful for my parents' kosher home for many reasons, but one of the most important was the lesson in mindfulness that came early in life. Before food or drink entered my mouth, I had to pause for at least a moment to ask, "Is this kosher?" That meant I had to stop, read a label, maybe talk to a waitress or chef, or perhaps pack my meal. The donut fried in lard, the cheeseburger, and the bacon never met my lips. At the time, I only thought about the Kashrut rules, but the gift that came with that mindfulness was better health. Kosher laws have always been, in part, both a way to honor God but also to honor our bodies.

In our modern society, however, kosher may not always equal healthy. Obesity, cancer, heart disease, diabetes, and dementia appear as common, or more common, in observant communities as in the general public. Who does not know of at least one prominent synagogue member lost to the community far before their expected years? I know many, and the loss was great. Diets heavy in meat, cream sauces, butter, and sugary sweets may all be kosher but cannot be considered healthy. That is where *Secrets of a Kosher Girl* comes in. To fully honor G-d and our amazing bodies, it takes an awareness of the laws of Kashrut interpreted in a modern view of nutritional balance, food additives, hormones, antibiotics, and calories. Beth Warren has the training, experience, and programs to take us to Mt. Sinai and beyond for our health.

Ms. Warren's 21-day program to weight loss and exercise is a refreshing spin on Kashrut and one you should take seriously. We eat too much of everything and certainly too much added sugars, trans and saturated fats, and calories, with inadequate fruit and vegetable intake. Her emphasis on whole foods, not from highly processed sources, is a path to the promised land of better health and less dependence on medications. It is a well-kept secret that many chronic diseases like heart disease, obesity, adult diabetes, and high blood pressure can be reversed by a whole foods diet rich in nourishing fruits and vegetables. Let's not keep that a secret anymore. Take part in the 21-day program from the Kosher Girl and enjoy better health and the *simcha* of feeling good every day.

*Joel Kahn, MD, is a plant-based kosher cardiologist who has launched a campaign to prevent one million heart attacks through healthy living. He teaches early detection, prevention, and reversal of heart disease. Dr.Kahn is the founder of the Kahn Center for Cardiac Longevity. He is a graduate Summa Cum Laude from the University of Michigan School of Medicine and is a Professor of Medicine. His books,* The Whole Heart Solution, *and* Dead Execs Don't Get Bonuses, *are both #1 bestsellers. He is co-owner of GreenSpace Cafe in Ferndale with his son Daniel. His PBS special,* The Whole Heart Solution, *is a pledge show now.*

# The Inception of a Kosher Girl

"All beginnings are hard."

—MEKHILTA YITRO

"Remember that while it can be hard to start to change, with effort
and practice, things do get easier. Keeping this in mind can help us
over the initial discomfort of trying something new."[1]

*K*osher girl. It's a title that elevates me to superhero status. I envision
myself standing on top of the Kotel, the Western Wall, in Jerusalem,
Israel with a cape flapping in the breeze, dressed in a blue and white
uniform. The outfit is a modest skirt that flows past my knees in the
country's signature colors and the shirt's collar reaches above my collar-
bone with sleeves that end below my elbows. Being a kosher girl is a
result of my genetics, a way of life I inherited by being born Jewish. The
kosher world shines meaning to my life and life to my soul. The kosher
girl is a term that reveals my inherent extraordinary power of keeping
a kosher diet, because committing to a kosher lifestyle sometimes
requires superhuman strength. My mission is to transform the purpose
of following a kosher lifestyle not just for spiritual reasons, but also to
promote health in everyone, regardless of religion (see the sidebar on
page xxi, "5 Ways Being Kosher Can Help Anyone, Not Just Jews").

## DAILY PRACTICES ON MY KOSHER GIRL'S DIET

- Mindful meditations every morning and at meal/snack times.
- Eat three satisfying meals and two delicious snacks of clean kosher whole foods that you will be preparing.
- Drink about 8–11 cups of approved drinks.
- Exercise at least 30–60 minutes of approved routines most days.

When I became a registered dietitian-nutritionist (RDN), I discovered a way to direct my life as a kosher girl along with its path of discipline and focus, benefitting my mind and body. Through my Jewish upbringing and specialty in weight loss in my private practice, I have found there are useful techniques that come with kosher living that can help you overcome the barriers inhibiting short and long-term weight loss success, whether Jewish or not. The kosher diet is not simply about the foods you can and cannot eat, but the equally powerful spiritual component that will help keep you mindful. This spiritual component can ease stress and teach critical behaviors associated with weight loss (see the sidebar on page xv, "What Is Kosher?").

Following a kosher lifestyle and a kosher diet can set the stage for helping you lose weight and keep it off when combined with a proven strategy of eating fewer processed and more "clean foods," more often. My diet uniquely integrates ancient kosher practices, including spiritual and standard rules of kosher law, with a nutritionally balanced, scientifically sound strategy utilizing a whole foods approach. My patients who follow this diet typically average 6 to 11 pounds of weight loss from fat, sustain or build muscle, and feel improvements in mood, energy, and other metrics including cholesterol and blood sugar—all in just 21 days.

## My Life on a Diet—and As an Expert

Although the weight loss situation may seem hopeless to many, I developed my kosher girl's diet as a way to help you achieve *true* weight loss and improvements in overall health without the false promises and unsustainable results of fad diets. Although kosher food can be unhealthy if one overindulges or if it's created with highly processed

## WHAT IS KOSHER?

- KOSHER: In Hebrew, "Kashrus," from the root kosher (or "kasher"), means suitable and/or "pure," thus ensuring fit for consumption. The laws of Kashrus include comprehensive legislation concerning permitted and forbidden foods.[39]
- CLEAN EATING: A concept that stresses eating whole, less processed foods.
- KOSHER CLEANSE: A way of eating and living that boosts overall health by combining the strategy to eat whole, less processed foods more often with ancient principles of a kosher diet to overcome weight loss barriers for short and long-term success.

ingredients, I found a way to utilize it properly to lose weight. Over time, I came to the enlightened realization that if a person can successfully keep kosher the way it was intended, keeping healthy should seamlessly fit together like bagels and lox.

It wasn't until I began grappling with weight loss and bearing witness as a registered dietitian to the struggles my clients face when trying to lose weight successfully and sustainably that I recognized the helpful link between keeping kosher and keeping healthy.

When I was growing up, food was the center of, well...everything. Judaism emphasizes celebratory events such as the weekly Sabbath, holidays, and social functions. What all these celebrations have in common is—you guessed it—food. As a result, within the Jewish culture, you will find delicious and abundantly served dishes created from sacred recipes passed with boasting pride from one generation to the next. I've had to train myself how to enjoy the meals and the company at these events without overindulging.

Throughout my life, my weight was at least ten pounds over what was healthy, which meant I could not simply eat whatever I wanted. That meant turning down all my childhood favorites including Drake's®, Dr Pepper®, Rollo®, and Slurpee®. Although I was physically active, taking dance classes since the age of six, playing in Little League, and going to the gym with my dad throughout my high school years, I had to learn how to fuse my love for food and its emphasis in my culture with my desire to be fit and healthy. Happily, I discovered my goals were not mutually exclusive.

In my youth, I was the girl who loved to eat. I was often found in school at the lunch table eating someone else's leftover meal, lurking around the vending machines to mooch off of someone else's soda and cookies, or being the first, middle, and the last hand in a bag of chips meant for four or more friends. It would be an understatement to say my eating habits were simply because I enjoyed food. I savored every finger-licking flavor as if it were the last taste I would consume during my lifetime.

Later, during my college years, I began to learn about the power of food after taking an elective nutrition course. I subsequently lost twelve pounds on my own before my wedding the same year I took that class. I furthered my education by obtaining my Master of Science degree in Nutrition and by working with clients of all ages, ethnicities, and various health goals. Aside from weight loss, many patients were also looking to improve their medical conditions. I found that losing weight, or what some of us would call "being on a diet," can be safe, delicious, and realistic, while also benefiting our overall well-being.

The next stage of my career was counseling patients from diverse backgrounds in my private practice, Beth Warren Nutrition. I uncovered a commonality in the frustration of weight loss, where I often faced the request for a quick-start program with results that would last. I was not willing to recommend something I knew might work in the short term and not be sustainable or make someone feel better in the long run. This strategy is solely responsible for helping me slim down after a 44-pound weight gain during the pregnancies of each of my five children, and this is the strategy you will see is solely responsible for helping my clients.

I know that my personal experiences of weight loss struggles are not unique; I've met countless individuals who have struggled with the same issues. The sad story about following a heavily restricted and imbalanced fad diet may tell a tale of quick weight loss, but it will conclude with an equally quick weight regain and poor quality of life. Unfortunately, if weight loss occurs too rapidly, it is not from fat but mostly from water and muscle loss. Your results are short-lived, and it becomes harder to lose weight the next time around, suffocating you inside the destructive cycle of yo-yo dieting.

It boggled my mind as I got older and more educated in nutrition that people who keep kosher for religious reasons are capable of following the strict laws, yet some of those same people can't find that same discipline and importance to staying healthy. I was one of those people and looked to figure out the disconnect, seeking to bridge the gap by linking the steadfast promise to keeping kosher with the same level of commitment to stay healthy and lose weight. I discovered in many ways that it came down to priorities. A top priority growing up was and still is my religion. Keeping kosher wasn't simply a way to eat, it was a *mitzvah* (commandment) by G-d to follow. Once I realized that it was also a mitzvah to keep my body healthy (a lesson learned from *Ushmartem es Nafshosechem*, about which you will read more in chapter 1), it became a no-brainer that my health should be as high of a priority. Further, combining the mitzvah to keep kosher with the mitzvah to keep healthy hits a "double whammy" in my personal goals of accomplishing G-d's will. Because we don't attribute eating to a higher awareness beyond physicality, it becomes difficult to overcome the urges that cause you to eat in a way that promotes weight gain.

As most people know, following a diet is more than adhering to rules dictating what to eat. The inability to follow through with the protocol is a frustration that passes through the lips of many clients and the reason they come to my office in the first place, apparently realizing that various factors need to work in tandem for them to stick with a plan. In fact, I would argue that keeping a sustainable diet is about 50 percent mindset, 40 percent diet, and 10 percent fitness. Your mind controls your awareness of the physical and the spiritual, and the link between the two is critical.

In Judaism, the intense desire to eat unhealthy foods even when you feel you have a stronger desire to eat healthily and lose weight can be a form of "yetzer harah," otherwise known as "evil inclination." The concept of the evil inclination can be any experience that presents an obstacle in life that you must work hard to overcome. Think of the common analogy of the good angel/bad angel perched on one's shoulders guiding life choices. Because it is a good deed, or mitzvah, to keep your body fit and healthy then the obstacle is intensely fierce in its opposition and works hard to convince you to make poor food choices and excuses not to exercise. However, a beautiful thought in Judaism is that G-d only puts obstacles in our path that we have the potential to overcome. (There is a dash in G-d because in Judaism, it is believed sacred to write out G-d). Once you become successful in removing the stumbling block, actual personal growth occurs.

Achieving your weight loss goals may feel impossible and take more work and dedication to be successful, but ultimately there is trust that you will make it to the other side of the struggle with the right plan. Once you reach the end of your 21-day journey, the accomplishment will be extra meaningful and sustainable because you overcame your strong desires to quit and transformed your entire mindset and lifestyle about healthy eating and living.

## PEARL'S STORY

*Beth Warren is a very personable and knowledgeable nutritionist. I partici-pated with a friendly group of people and completed her 21-Day Kosher Cleanse.*

*We ate a very balanced diet of whole foods. I was so excited that at the end I lost 10 pounds! I usually lose weight very slowly, so that was huge.*

*Beth taught me so much about eating a healthier way. I can't say I'm 100% a healthy eater, but I'd say I'm greatly improved over one year later. I no longer bring white rice, white potatoes, or white pasta into the house! That's a huge change for this pasta eating person! Fresh fruits and salads and veggies are a solid part of my day. My favorite store is Trader Joe's.*

*I have continued to lose weight since I've last seen Beth over one year ago. I wear a dress size that makes me pinch myself. I truly thought it couldn't happen without weight loss surgery. Beth also introduced me to wearing a fitness tracker. I don't take 10,000 steps a day, but I walk or use the treadmill and go to exercise classes too!*

*Thank you, Beth Warren!*

## Why This Will Work for You

My "aha" moment connected the ability to lose weight and keep it off with a more meaningful level of purpose and transformed my entire nutrition strategy. Religion aside, I seek to work on the principles of keeping kosher that anyone can benefit from so that clients finally overcome many barriers to weight loss. As much as I guarantee short-term weight and fat loss results, especially with this 21-day plan, my goal is to build a foundation in that period so sustainable results occur naturally. My heart breaks each time a client comes to me for the first time and explains his or her struggle with not only weight loss but keeping off lost weight. I feel deeply for their disappointment after following a deprivation diet for some time only to be in a worse state both physically and emotionally sometime later. My plan celebrates eating whole kosher foods while automatically setting the stage for building habits and eating behaviors so that one can feel motivated to keep up the lifestyle and maintain weight loss.

*My diet philosophy is simple.* I combine my unique spin on changing negative eating behavior by using substantiated methods already inherent in the kosher lifestyle with proven ways to boost metabolism by eating clean, less processed foods. There is no one bad food or food group on my plan. Instead, I rotate food choices, especially carbohydrate sources, to promote an anti-inflammatory diet that curbs cravings and keeps you satisfied, while aiding in weight loss and better overall health.

While reading this book, you will discover my secrets to successful weight loss that lasts. I purposefully calculate each method, type of food, time of eating, food combination, and kosher requirements. You are not doing something on my diet that serves only to make your life more difficult. Each food and nutrition recommendation provides a ripple effect that wards off the monsters lurking in the shadows waiting to scare you into diet failure.

## What You Can Expect

To better understand my book, I have summarized each of the four parts I have developed for my program:

In Part One, I explain how you can adequately prepare your mind, body, and pantry to follow the diet successfully. Methods for establishing a strong spiritual connection inherent in a kosher lifestyle, to prepare the mind to help you successfully lose weight, are included in chapter one. Chapter two explains the role of physical activity, not only as a critical component in health and weight loss nowadays, but as an endorsed concept since biblical times. The goal of chapter three is to create the simplest shopping experience at any supermarket with tips on how to navigate the aisles for both clean and kosher foods, including detailed weekly shopping lists for the foods needed for each week of the diet.

In Part Two, I provide everything you need to be aware of while following the diet, the critical nutrition guidelines that act as the foundation of the plan, including information about a kosher diet as it applies to the 21-day program.

Part Three spells out the actual diet program: a 21-day breakdown of meal plans, recipes, and daily fitness goals, with my favorite kosher motivational quotes to keep you inspired along the way.

Part Four provides recommendations on how to maintain your results.

*Secrets of a Kosher Girl* takes you on an invigorating journey with reliable results of fat loss along with boosts in energy, muscle mass, mood, and behavior. My diet has not only scientific data to prove its effectiveness, but also inspirational real-life testimonials.

Frequently, my clients realized they hadn't achieved the weight loss they expected or that weight loss is not the only indicator of how successful they were while being on a different diet. Important factors such as how they feel and how physically fit they look are key indicators of successful dieting. So too is the critical aspect of whether the way they were eating is a way they can sustain, and therefore keep the weight off. Ultimately, after just one consultation with me, they discovered that whatever they thought they knew about weight loss was incomplete at best and wrong at worst. They discovered, and you will learn, that my diet is motivating and realistic. *Secrets of a Kosher Girl* is filled with practical tools you need to help you lose weight at a more rapid pace than with a standard meal plan and improve your wellbeing while providing you with the knowledge necessary for maintaining the beneficial results beyond the 21 days.

## New Research and Credibility

My kosher girl's diet is different because it is a guide for life, providing strategies and proven tips for getting on track to a whole new healthy kosher lifestyle. Studies show that participants who ate a whole foods

## 5 WAYS BEING KOSHER CAN HELP ANYONE, NOT JUST JEWS

1. Kosher clearly distinguishes types of food including dairy, meat, and "pareve" (neither dairy nor meat) on packages, simplifying food choices for those who cannot tolerate them, who are allergic, or who are vegan.
2. It teaches you to not trust a product based on what it claims on the package, but the need to delve into the ingredients used and the processing methods. By digging deeper into how a product is made and reading food labels, you can make a more educated, cleaner, healthier choice of foods you purchase so that it helps weight loss.
3. The guidelines and laws establish self-discipline and awareness, two attributes that can help achieve and sustain weight loss.
4. The focus on spirituality and self-awareness in your mind and body, recognizing that your body is a holy vessel that should be treated with care through fitness and healthy eating.
5. The daily practices that reinforce mindful eating and positive self-affirmations that lead to sustainable changes in your overall health, not just weight loss.

diet metabolized foods 50 percent faster than those who ate processed foods, which can lead to more rapid weight loss. Behavioral modifications inherent within a kosher lifestyle are also shown to be critical to weight loss efforts by the *Food and Nutrition Report*.[2] Keeping kosher requires self-discipline and mindfulness, making the diet more likely to be successful. Along with sustainable weight loss, my diet results in fat loss, a shrunken waist and hip circumference, and an increase in lean muscle mass. Every result correlates to a decrease in morbidity and mortality rate, an improved quality of life, and a better looking you, regardless of your age or how long you've been struggling with your weight.

## The Bottom Line

My diet uniquely uses kosher guidelines and spiritual components to change food choices and behaviors that act as a barrier to successful weight loss, creating a healthier, easier, and faster weight loss during the 21 days. The diet takes into account an array of lifestyle factors you may experience, which makes the program realistic at any level. Enticing kosher meal plans targeting weight loss, detailed shopping lists of kosher foods that can be found in most supermarkets or online, easy-to-follow recipes, and authentic testimonials and motivational biblical quotes all help you get on the path of healthy living. My kosher girl's diet is a refreshing spin on weight loss strategies proven to work. It will motivate you to finally lose weight and keep it off while feeling less restricted and healthier overall.

*Secrets of a Kosher Girl* was specifically created because it is the answer to:

▶ Finding a quick-start program to facilitate weight loss using kosher guidelines combined with a whole food strategy proven to work for anyone.

▶ The struggle with emotional barriers to losing weight and keeping it off using the spiritual connection associated with a kosher diet.

▶ Restrictive fad diets that are ephemeral at best.

▶ A safe and efficient strategy to dieting.

▶ Finding a lifestyle-oriented plan.

▶ Not only weight loss, but better overall health and relief of certain health conditions.

▶ Solidifying the mind-body connection to improve overall quality of life.

## MEET CHAIM

*My name is Chaim Tabak, age 30. When I was young, I was cute and very skinny. But like every kid, I loved eating whatever I could get a hold of including cakes, candies and all the 'goodies' that a kid can imagine.*

*As I grew older and reached the age of Bar Mitzvah (13 years old), I also grew in size and became chubby. But it didn't stop there. As I went on in life, I kept indulging in the 'goodies' figuring that it was okay, and grew bigger. With every visit to the doctor, I got the same warning—that I am overweight. I started to hate going to the doctor but did nothing about what he told me.*

*By the time I got married, I was over 200 pounds. Shortly after that, I had (naturally) gained even more weight since I was eating lots of cakes, pastries, fried and fast foods, with not much healthful food. Approximately at the age of 24, the doctor told me that my cholesterol was too high and put me on medication. Still not wanting to do anything about my weight, and never doing any exercise, (I have always said, 'You live once, I want to enjoy it'), I kept eating the wrong foods thinking this is best for me and eventually it hit me. By the time I reached 30 years old, I had realized that I was on cholesterol medication for about six years. In the last six years, I also suffered from back pain, which my doctor told me was related to my obesity and that I needed to lose weight. I noticed that it got harder for me to get around or go upstairs due to being obese and lazy. It hit me that diabetes runs in the family and that the longer I waited, the harder the battle to lose weight would be. I didn't want to take pills and medications for the rest of my life! Thinking of all that scared me, and I decided that the time had come for me to start losing weight and be a healthier person.*

*The first step I did was cut down on cakes and fried food, and I started cycling a bit, but it didn't help much. So I looked into a nutritionist, and I am glad I met with Beth Warren. When I did, my life changed forever for the better. Beth explained to me the differences between food categories, when, what, and how much to eat, and put together a kosher whole foods menu that I was to follow, and I did! Beth also encouraged and motivated me to exercise more often, and I did! The results? I went off my cholesterol medication; my back pain decreased, I lost a whopping 70 pounds, and went from a pants size 46 down to size 34. I feel like a free man now by not being tied to any meds and being able to walk, jump, and run as I please.*

*To sum it up, what I did was instead of going on a temporary crash diet, I permanently changed my lifestyle and got used to eating healthfully and exercising on a daily basis. That is what made me lose my weight and is helping me to keep it off in a healthful manner. I now don't eat all the types of food I used to, and to be honest, I don't even feel like I'm missing out on any of it. I enjoy a delicious bowl of salad with some protein rather than an egg roll or any fast food items. It's been four years, and I've kept the weight off. I live much more happily now and enjoy life much more.*

*Thank You, Beth Warren, for your support, motivation, and guidance to a better and healthier lifestyle!*

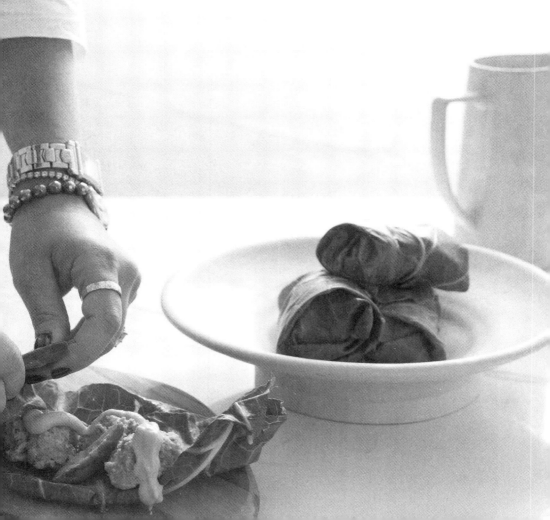

# Part One
# GET PREPPED

*"And you shall eat and be satisfied,
and you shall bless Hashem, your G–d,
for the good land which He has given you."*
—DEUTERONOMY 8:10

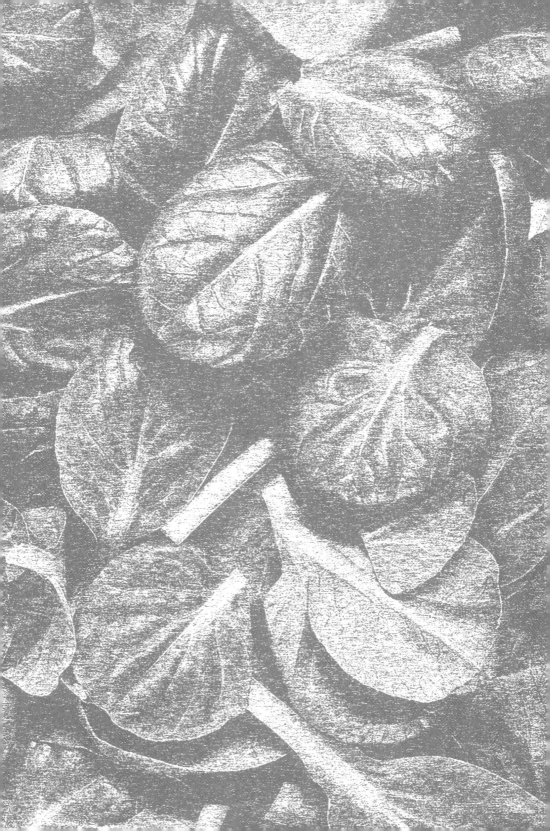

CHAPTER 1

# Mind Over Matter

"Looking upon leads to awareness.
Awareness leads to action."

—*TALMUD*, MENACHOT 43B

## Why Mindful Eating Leads to Weight Loss

You may be wondering why I am stressing the importance of mindful eating in a diet book. The reason is that you can neither diet successfully nor keep off the hard-earned weight loss without first and foremost working on your mind. It's a component lacking in most weight loss programs and the reason why dieters struggle to reach and maintain weight loss goals. I also aim to make my diet as effortless as possible. Research suggests that when you eat slower and more thoughtfully, you may steer away from highly processed food and unhealthy choices, making it easier for you to stick with the whole foods built into my plan.[3]

Ultimately, I want you to fall in love with the food you are eating on my kosher girl's diet. Mindfulness can help with your enjoyment of healthy food as well. A random-controlled study included 150 binge eaters to compare a mindfulness-based therapy to a standard psycho-educational treatment and a control group. Both active treatments produced declines in binging and depression, but the mindfulness-based therapy seemed to help people enjoy their food more and have less sense of struggle about controlling their eating. Those who meditated more during the study (both at mealtimes and throughout

3

the day) got more out of the program, a similar practice of saying blessings at meals on a kosher diet that you will read about in this chapter.

Mindfulness is also shown to reduce stress. Thus, when following mindfulness techniques on my diet and applying them to your eating habits, you will feel less stressed out about your choices. This practice will help you stay in control and guide you to make healthy decisions the whole way through. And since stress is often at the root of overeating, mindfulness seems to make us eat better meals, which means you will happily stick with my plan.

Mindful practices like meditation are shown to improve health, medical problems such as high blood pressure and gastrointestinal difficulties, lessen pain and sickness to a significant part because they reduce stress, according to a *Time* magazine report.[4] These findings are a major reason why my diet not only results in weight loss, but better overall health. In this chapter, I will share the spiritual foundation you need to achieve to be successful on my kosher girl's diet.

## Breaking Down the Weight Loss Barriers

We can all admit that one reason for regaining weight is that we fall back into bad habits. Mindless eating is one of the sabotaging behaviors that cause weight gain and is a reason behind dieting failure. If you're unsure whether or not you present the ways of a mindless eater, ask yourself the following questions:

1.  Do I tend to continue eating even though I am full?
2.  Do I eat when I'm emotional, even if I'm not hungry?
3.  Do I "pick" at foods, or "munch"?
4.  Do I tend to make judgments on myself when I overeat?
5.  Do I multitask when I eat?
6.  Do I always eat everything on my plate?
7.  Do I eat fast, hardly chewing my food?
8.  Do I not appreciate the way food is nourishing my body while I am eating?

If you answered "yes" to any of these questions, you likely engage in some form of mindless eating that will ultimately be your dieting pitfall. Don't fret: You are going to use the spiritual awareness built into a kosher diet to achieve stronger self-control and discipline when faced with foods off the diet plan. My goal is to show you how I found a close link between the mind and body by keeping kosher and help you find your mindful connection. Once you successfully conquer your mind by emulating principles behind keeping kosher, you will experience weight loss.

## How to Cultivate a Spiritual Conversation

Eating is mundane. The behavior is instinctive because we need to eat every day for survival. It is easy, therefore, for eating to be mindless—an act we do without thought that contributes to weight gain. The act of food preparation alone that you will read about in the next chapter, integral to my kosher girl's diet, will cause you to eat more mindfully and appreciate the food in front of you. In Judaism, another way to keep mindful of what you are eating is the act of saying blessings. By saying a blessing, you are forced to pause a few moments in front of the food without eating it, recite a few words to yourself, and only then recognize what you are about to eat. By those simple actions of setting an intention, you transform the ordinariness of eating into a holy experience. Eating at home, with friends, at work, while celebrating or hanging out, the act transcends the monotonous into an exciting experience to which you pay attention every time.

Anyone can find his or her way to adopt this practice. From Christianity, to Buddhism, to Judaism, saying a blessing before a meal is not exclusive to any one type of religion or movement. A simple difference is that Jews who keep kosher do not say a blessing on the meal as a whole, but take it a step further by reciting one on each specific type of food category present and in a particular order. I adopted the art of making a mindful connection before eating through blessings in my kosher girl's diet. By giving more attention to each food from reciting numerous blessings, you elevate mindfulness, intention, and appreciation of your meal to another level.

Regardless of religion, you can discover your way to establish the mindful connection over food. To find your ultimate blessing, it may help to understand more about the Hebrew word for blessing, "*brachah.*" The six blessings for different food groups (see the "Blessings in Judaism" sidebar below), all start by acknowledging G-d as the source of sustenance and express gratitude to Him for providing it to us. The words begin with, *"Blessed are You, Lord our G-d, King of the universe..."* When I make a *brachah*, the action sets me up to be mindfully aware of the food I am about to consume. You can adopt my way, or you can set your intention for what makes you feel grateful before eating. Whether it be the soil of nature, the farmers, or your supermarket, on my kosher girl's diet you should verbalize intent and simple thanks before eating so that your mind transcends outside of the meal for a moment and as a result, fosters mindful awareness of what you are eating.

## EXAMPLES OF BLESSINGS IN JUDAISM ON EACH FOOD[5]

Six different *brochot* (blessings) correspond to the various food categories. They belong to the type of blessing called *bircat ha'nehenin* (blessings of pleasure), which are required to recite before we derive physical pleasure from G–d's creations.

Before partaking of any food, a *brachah rishonah* (preceding blessing), is said. There are six different blessings, each beginning with the same words, BA-RUCH A-TAH A-DO-NOI ELO-HAI-NU ME-LECH HA-O-LAM, Blessed are You, L–rd our G–d, King of the Universe, concluding with a few words related to the type of food eaten. Following are the food groups with examples for each group and a transliteration and translation of the Hebrew blessing for each.

1. On bread, bagels, challah, matzah, pita, and rolls made from any of these five grains: wheat, barley, rye, oats, or spelt:
   BA-RUCH A-TAH A-DO-NOI
   ELO-HAI-NU ME-LECH HA-O-LAM
   HA-MO-TZI LE-CHEM MIN HA-A-RETZ.
   Blessed are You, L–rd our G–d, King of the Universe,
   Who brings forth bread from the Earth.

2. On cakes, cereals, cookies, cupcakes, doughnuts, and pasta, if made of one or more of the five grains listed under the first blessing:
   BA-RUCH A-TAH A-DO-NOI
   ELO-HAI-NU ME-LECH HA-O-LAM
   BO-RAI MI-NAI ME-ZO-NOT.
   Blessed are You, L–rd our G–d, King of the Universe,
   Who creates various kinds of sustenance.

3. On wine and grape juice:
   BA-RUCH A-TAH A-DO-NOI
   ELO-HAI-NU ME-LECH HA-O-LAM
   BO-RAI PRI HA-GA-FEN.
   Blessed are You, L–rd our G–d, King of the Universe,
   Who creates the fruit of the vine.

4. For all fruits from trees, such as apples, oranges, and peaches, even if
   these fruits are dried; also grapes, raisins, and all nuts (except peanuts,
   which is a legume):
   BA-RUCH A-TAH A-DO-NOI
   ELO-HAI-NU ME-LECH HA-O-LAM
   BO-RAI PRI HA-AITZ.
   Blessed are You, L–rd our G–d, King of the Universe,
   Who creates the fruit of the tree.

5. For all vegetables and greens from the ground, peanuts, legumes, and
   some fruits such as bananas, melons, and pineapples:
   BA-RUCH A-TAH A-DO-NOI
   ELO-HAI-NU ME-LECH HA-O-LAM
   BO-RAI PRI HA-A-DA-MAH.
   Blessed are You, L–rd our G–d, King of the Universe,
   Who creates the fruit of the Earth.

6. For candy, dairy, eggs, fish, liquids, meat, mushrooms, and everything
   else not included in the first five blessings:
   BA-RUCH A-TAH A-DO-NOI
   ELO-HAI-NU ME-LECH HA-O-LAM
   SHE-HA-KOL NI-H'YAH BI-D'VA-RO.
   Blessed are You, L–rd our G–d, King of the Universe,
   by Whose word all things came to be.

NOTE: The above blessings apply to foods in their basic form; however,
the blessings may vary when the form is changed through processing, or
when foods are combined.

## Keeping Mindful Beyond the Meal

In Judaism, we once again remember G-d as the ultimate source of our sustenance after eating, as instructed in the Bible, *"And you shall eat and be satisfied, and you shall bless Hashem, your G-d, for the good land which He has given you."* (Deuteronomy 8:10) This particular command stipulates a blessing after the meal, not before, and according to chabad.org, is a custom still honored today by observant Jews in the *Birkat Hamazon* (Grace After Meals).

The meditation after a meal further emphasizes mindful eating practices. By taking those extra moments, you relax in one place and allow the food to settle in your stomach. The time of introspection creates an opportunity to evaluate how the meal made you feel: satisfied, full, stuffed? You can gain a lot of information in the hour after you've eaten a meal. While being on my kosher girl's diet, pay attention: do you feel sick, stuffed, or tired? Are you satisfied? Are you still hungry? In my diet's Wellness Planner, you will note the answers to these questions and find patterns as to which foods and meals work best for you.

Try this guided meditation after eating each meal and snack on my meal plan:

▶ Did you like the taste of the food you ate?

▶ Do you like how the food made you feel after you ate it?

▶ Do you like how it made you feel in your mind? Do you feel guilty, happy, pleased, etc.?

▶ Do you feel more energized or sleepier after eating?

▶ Do you feel satisfied, full, or stuffed?

▶ What did you learn about what you just ate and how would that affect your future choice of foods or meal composition? For example, was it too heavy for a particular type of carbohydrate such as brown rice? Would you prefer a starchy vegetable such as a sweet potato next time? Does that make your belly feel less stuffed? Would that cause you to feel less guilty about eating it?

As you can see, there are a lot of questions to ask yourself after eating. The answers bring you closer to the root of understanding which foods make your dietetic clock tick. Your body communicates without words, similar to a pet or an infant who cannot articulate exactly what it wants. You will learn to listen to the subtle cues it's trying to tell you and act accordingly. By understanding how your body speaks, you will learn not to ignore it with constant daily pressures, such as a deadline you have for a project at work, that fight to take priority in your consciousness.

When digesting food, a complex series of hormonal signals between the gut and the nervous system occurs, and it seems to take about 20 minutes for the brain to register satiety and fullness. If you eat too fast, satiety may occur *after* overeating instead of *before*. Additionally, while you are eating you are often distracted by activities like driving or typing, and that may slow down or stop digestion similar to how the "fight or flight" response does. If we're not digesting well, we may be missing out on the full nutritive value of some of the food we're consuming, according to The Harvard School of Public Health.

Not surprisingly, research supports the benefits of mindfulness on satiety cues since it is shown to sharpen a person's ability to recognize internal cues that signal hunger and fullness. Similar mindful meditations are naturally within Judaism and the kosher diet. I once heard a story from a rabbi who had diabetes and who overcame his addiction to salted potato chips that were hurting him by repeating the mantra of *"ushmartem es nafshosechem"* or "protect your body." The quote is a commandment by G-d written in the Bible that the rabbi adapted as a form of meditation when faced with unhealthy foods. The rabbi understood that consuming the chips was endangering his life and that was a prohibition by a higher power. He could not succeed in resisting the junk foods for himself, but when he made the spiritual connection with mindful meditation, he was able to overcome the unhealthy urge to eat it.

## Mindfulness Will Help Your Craving on My Diet

By advocating clean foods that curb cravings on my plan, you will not have as much desire to munch on junk foods, allowing you to finally release the baggage you *shlep* along with you during and after weight loss attempts. Mindful eating is another way to help you curb cravings. A lot of your urge to eat salty or sweet foods comes from remembering the experience of what they feel like in your mouth. Studies show you acti-vate the same areas of the brain as you do when you eat the food.[6] That's why it is so hard to resist plowing through a bag of potato chips you love when it's in front of you. But guess what? Mindful eating disrupts the automatic reaction by reducing the appeal of unhealthy foods.

Esther Papies, a social psychologist studying self-regulation and health behaviors at the University of Glasgow in the UK, says that the trick is to think of your food craving as nothing more than a mere thought that's fleeting—kind of like a soap bubble that will disappear as soon as you touch it. Pop the craving as soon as it pops up in your mind.

## Working Mindfulness into My Kosher Girl's Diet

How can you work on the art of mindful eating? Pay attention to the colors, aromas, flavors, and textures of your food during the 21 days on my diet. Chew slowly, get rid of distractions like TV or reading, and learn to cope with guilt and anxiety about food. Eating on my diet will become such a positive experience that you are feeling happy and encouraged despite the opposite feelings instinctively arising with the declaration, "I'm going on a diet." On the Wellness Planner, you will note all details of the experience of eating, not solely what foods you ate.

Even though the nature of a kosher diet incorporates meditations as a way to stay mindful, you will also write a detailed food-mood diary in the form of a Wellness Planner, which is a proven method to help keep you aware and is also an independent factor that facilitates weight loss. A Wellness Planner records every bite you consume but should answer questions such as, "How does this meal smell?" and "What are its colors and textures?" Surprising to researchers of one study, the people who used a food-mood diary surpassed the group that solely relied on medi-tation to maintain their weight loss. While following my 21-day plan, I recommend you write a Wellness Planner (see the sample on page 240) to keep you fully engaged in the diet and with yourself. My goal is not only for you to achieve weight loss in the present moment, but have you maintain your hard-earned results.

## REAL-LIFE KOSHER GIRL

*Hi. My name is Leah. I am 46 years old, and I am blessed with six children. As I got older, and with each child, I began to put on weight. It came to a point where I felt the need to take charge of the steady increase and follow a diet to lose weight. Little did I know that when I met with Beth I would experience something so far beyond simply discussing what food to eat. The aspect of her diet that really hit home and allowed me to lose 20 pounds is the spiritual component that keeps me mindful. I wouldn't explain to others that I'm on a diet. I simply convey that I am sincerely focused on my foods and mindfully make choices on what I know I really want to eat at that moment. I attack each eating situation, whether with my kids on Saturday night, a typical tempting time for overeating, at events, or simply a standard night of dinner where I may have made not as healthy options, and I ask myself the questions, "Is this what I really want right now?" and "Is eating this going to make me feel happy afterward?" If the answer is yes, I mindfully treat myself to a small portion, I enjoy it, and then I put it completely out of my mind and move forward on my more healthful path. It's that sense of freedom while still being in control that allows me to be able to stick to the plan. Plus, the added spiritual fact that I know that what I am doing for my body is for the better helps keep me mindful.*

*Now that you know my story, here is my message to you:*

Dear Readers,

Let's define "spiritual dieting."

The reason so many people get frustrated after attempting weight loss is that there is an aspect of knowledge that is missing.

That is a belief in the togetherness of our emotional health as well as our physical well-being and spiritual status.

When we bless the food we eat, let's make it be a reason to smile. Besides for feeling grateful for the delicious taste we are about to experience, we will take a moment to focus on the fact that can give our souls the nourishment it craves.

Let's do it for ourselves, our families and friends, and last but not least, for our overall well-being.

Enjoy!

**HUNGER AND FULLNESS SCALE**

| Rating | | Physical Sensation |
|---|---|---|
| | 1 | Starvation, need to eat now, hunger pains, shaky, light-headed |
| | 2 | Slight pain in stomach, hard to concentrate, lack of energy |
| Ideal Zone | 3 | Beginning of physical signs of hunger, stomach growling sometimes |
| | 4 | Could eat if it were suggested |
| | 5 | Neutral |
| | 6 | Satisfied |
| | 7 | Feel food in stomach |
| | 8 | Stomach sticks out |
| | 9 | Bloated, clothes feel tight, sleepy and drained |
| | 10 | Definitely full, stomach uncomfortable, no energy, physically weak |

Source: Based on NEMO team health.qld.gov.au/nutrition
© The State of Queensland (Queensland Health) 1996–2016

# How to Achieve Mindfulness Each Day of the Diet

I know mindful eating may seem easier to say than to do, which is why a kosher lifestyle implements ways to reawaken the mindfully spiritual connection with daily practices. On the diet in part 3, you begin each day with a mantra and meditation to help focus the mind. Before eating each food, you will say your form of blessing or motivational quote, getting you centered and focused.

You can try these simple tips from Harvard Health that may help you get started on your path toward finding your own mindfulness.[7]

- ▸ Set your kitchen timer to 20 minutes, and take that time to eat a meal.
- ▸ Try eating with your non-dominant hand. If you're a righty, hold your fork in your left hand when lifting food to your mouth.
- ▸ Use chopsticks if you don't regularly use them.

▶ Eat silently for five minutes, thinking about what it took to produce that meal, from the sun's rays to the farmer, to the grocer, to the cook.

▶ Take small bites and chew well.

▶ Before opening the fridge or cabinet, take a breath and ask yourself, "Am I really hungry?"

▶ Do something else, like reading or going on a short walk.

▶ Put your cellphone down and away from the table.

When you practice mindful behavior, you will foster a strong mind-body connection and become completely in tune with your wants and needs that will aid in both short and long-term weight loss success.

## What to Expect in the Next Chapter

It's interesting that we have not yet begun to discuss actual food. We make the mistake of jumping over the basic foundation to successful weight loss—the powerful mind, which is a unique step to my diet plan. Now that you've established a solid mindset and techniques to find your spiritual connection capable of overcoming any mindless diet sabotage, you can learn about the food on my diet in the next chapter.

# CHAPTER 2

# The Sweat of Your Brow

"Great is our physical demand. We need a healthy body. We dealt much with soulfulness; we forgot the holiness of the body. We neglected the physical health and strength; we forgot that we have holy flesh; no less than holy spirit..."

—RAV ABRAHAM ISAAC KOOK (1865–1935),
AN INFLUENTIAL RABBI OF THE TWENTIETH CENTURY

Aside from mindful exercises, a kosher life of physical activity is an integral part of Judaism. Because our physical self protects our spiritual souls, there is a mitzvah to keep those bodies fit. Unfortunately, many people do not deem fitness as high of a priority as they should. Maimonides, a medieval Sephardic Jewish philosopher and respected doctor, highlighted the dangers of lack of fitness ages ago when he wrote, "Anyone who lives a sedentary life and does not exercise...even if he eats good foods and takes care of himself according to proper principles, all his days will be painful ones and his strength will wane."[8]

It is also no secret today in modern science that exercise is great for overall health. Studies show fitness helps in preventing cancer, type 2 diabetes, and other diseases along with improving cognitive health, aging, and mood.[9] But does exercise help weight loss? Believe it or not, the answer is a conditional yes, and only if fitness is performed in the right balance with the goal to lose weight along with what and when you are eating. A study in the *American Journal of Clinical Nutrition* (AJCN) found, "Incorporating exercise training into obesity treatment had led to 'inconsistent results,'" while other studies found it helped.[10]

In this chapter, you will learn how to exercise to promote weight loss and target fat loss while enhancing mindfulness and self-awareness on my diet.

## Thinking Quality Over Quantity

The days when we felt the only way to exercise for weight loss was to jump for hours like kangaroos amped up on caffeine are gone. Today, studies are painting a more cautionary picture. The AJCN research warned that after exercising we may compensate with more sedentary activities and potentially counteract the benefits on weight, explaining: "The increased energy expenditure obtained by training may be offset by a decrease in non-training physical activities."[7] However, inactivity is not the only way to compensate for fitness; you can be doing it with your food too. The issue is this: While you burn calories through exercise, which has the potential to yield weight loss, you also stimulate hunger. While you suppress your appetite during exercise, it can come back with a vengeance afterward when your hunger hormones surge and your satiety hormones drop. Because studies prove that you may eat more after too much intensive exercise whether because you are hungrier or compensate with food, you negate the calorie deficit you created and can potentially gain weight. Conclusions such as these suggest that over-exercising may contribute to weight gain, not coveted weight loss.

Of course, there are ways to use exercise to our advantage. The issue boils down to quantity versus quality fitness and its effects on your weight. Before bursting your fitness bubble, allow me to boast about the positives of implementing quality fitness for weight loss, and more specifically, fat versus muscle loss. Ultimately, we diet to look lean and fit. You do not end up looking the way you want after following a very rapid weight loss plan since you often lose loads of muscle. My diet promise is that you end up feeling and looking your best by sustaining or boosting muscle and losing fat on my fitness plan.

## My Life in Fitness

I am a fitness fan and enjoy switching up my routine. I love pushing my limits in the various regimes and discovering how I can conquer my mind to strengthen my body beyond what I thought it could do. The feeling is an empowering boost that motivates me to pursue my kosher clean eating regiment each day. It is a pet peeve of mine when I hear, "You do not have to exercise to lose weight." That ideology is completely missing the point of how fitness helps you in more ways with your weight loss efforts than changing the number on the scale. Exercise helps keep you motivated. Exercise helps keep you focused. Exercise helps you look fit, your ultimate reason for pursuing weight loss. Exercise builds your confidence. Finally, finding your exercise niche while following the diet allows you to develop a habit that will be a major player in maintaining your weight loss over time.

## Overcoming the True Obstacle: Time

I get asked when is the ideal time to exercise often. It's a question that is typically followed up with a personal one asking how I manage to fit fitness into my day. As an über-busy business owner, director of a private practice with multiple locations, staff members to manage, and responsibilities as a wife and mom of five young kids, my best answer is that time is what I manage to make of it.

If something is important to you, you will make time for it. The ability to prioritize fitness into the day is that simple in my mind. If I overthink how I am going to find the time, I won't be able to fit fitness into my day. There is no apparent "right time" in life when you have other commitments and priorities. You simply need to put your fitness as high of a priority as your other commitments. It gets a scheduled time and focused attention just like the other hundreds of things you need to do in a day.

Luckily, research validates my crazy schedule when it comes to fitting in my workout. Exercise is great to perform anytime you make it happen. On my kosher girl's diet, I set up the meal plan with scheduled meals and snacks that can technically support exercise at any time during the day (see the "21 Day Plan for Keeping Fit While Keeping Kosher" on page 253). However, Maimonides states that a person, "Should engage one's body and exert oneself in a sweat-producing task each morning." He again references the best time to exercise when he writes, "The best time for exercise is at the beginning of the day, upon awakening from sleep, and after the expulsion of the superfluities..."[11]

I often see with clients and myself that when we push off fitness, it becomes harder to push ourselves to do the activity. The mind and body will most likely be pulled in numerous directions over the course of the day, leaving our workout at the bottom of the totem pole.

On another note, people tend to get hungrier in the latter part of the day. As a result, the optional after dinner snack on my kosher girl's diet may not be enough to hold you off from eating until breakfast the next day. Before you think about it too hard, try making exercise a priority in your morning.

## What Exercise You Should Be Doing?

From boxing, hot yoga, Pilates on a mega reformer, Zumba, to training for half-marathons with my Team SBH*, I welcome just about any workout into my repertoire. It is fun getting swept up with excitement to challenge my mind and body while reveling in the results on my physical and emotional well-being. Although you do not have to become quite as enthusiastic about pursuing every degree of exercise recommended in the "Resources for Fitness" section, here are three workout regiments you can do on my kosher girl's diet for optimal results:

### Walking

Walking was part of the Jewish culture for centuries since it was thought then and is currently proven to be effective for establishing a healthy weight. In the Talmud (the body of Jewish civil and ceremonial law and legend comprising the *Mishnah and the Gemara*) tractate Shabbat, 41a states, *"Walking was felt to be beneficial to other organ systems; after meals one should perform some exercise; if one eats without walking four cubits after it, the food rots in the intestines and is not digested."* Additionally, on the Sabbath day, Saturday, a biblically ordained day of rest when forms of work including exercise are prohibited, walking is permitted: *"Walking on the Sabbath is not only permissible, but desirable."* (Tosefta Peah 4:10; Tosefta Shabbat 16:17).

---

* I act as the sports nutritionist for 300+ runners each year for a nonprofit organization, Sephardic Biker Holim.

Although oversimplified, the age-old theory "calories in equal calories out" would mean that walking should cause weight loss just as well as more cumbersome exercises because it also burns calories. Maimonides recommends exercise both in his *Code of Jewish Law* known as the *Mishneh Torah* and in his *Medical Aphorisms*, where he states, *"I, Maimonides, ascribe great importance to the regulation and maintenance of physical and mental health."* Interestingly, he too later stresses the harmful effects of excessively strenuous exercise, stating that, *"... walking, bathing, and gentle massage with rubbing oil suffices."*[12]

After the completion of the diet, walking will remain a part of your day and help keep the weight off. A study in the *Journal of the American Medical Association* followed the exercise habits of over 34,000 women and concluded that it took about an hour a day of moderate (3 mph walking) activity to maintain weight. This research supported the findings of the National Weight Control Registry, which reported that 90 percent of people who have successfully lost weight and kept it off exercise on average for an hour a day, and that can be from walking!

## Interval-Based Training

Throw down those dumbbells and pump some iron. A more time-efficient and proven way to lose fat and effectively exercise is to do high-intensity circuit training versus constant aerobics. The definition of short-term moderate-to-high-intensity exercise training, otherwise known as "HIIT," may mean bursts of more intensive exercise lasting between 30 seconds to three minutes, followed by recovery periods of as little as a few seconds or as long as 15 minutes. Personally, I love using a jump rope for my bursts of intensity and then various planks, lunges, and squats for my working recoveries. In addition to improving aerobic fitness, interval training can burn more calories quickly. Since most people who use time management as an excuse not to participate in fitness, HIIT workouts are an obvious choice. Additionally, there is evidence showing intervals trigger a mechanism that not only helps the body burn more fat, but possibly boost metabolism for some period after the workout ends.[13] For the already fit, the key to receiving benefits from a HIIT workout is to go hard during those intense periods. You know you are doing exercises correctly when you cannot carry on a conversation during the high intervals.

Studies show HIIT can induce modest body composition improvements in overweight and obese individuals without necessarily accompanying body-weight changes. One study stated HIIT and MICT (moderate interval circuit training) show similar effectiveness across all body composition measures, suggesting that HIIT may be a time-efficient component of weight management programs as well. HIIT three times per week for 15 weeks compared to the same frequency of standard exercise was associated with significant reductions in total body fat, subcutaneous leg and trunk fat, and insulin resistance in young women.[14] In my diet, with the combination of incorporating quality fat-burning foods into a regimented meal plan plus the HIIT component, we will achieve both weight loss and fat loss on the program that is also sustainable.

## Yoga

There is a story recorded about Rav Simhah Bunim of Przysucha, who arrived late for synagogue one Sabbath morning. When asked why he was late, he quoted from Pesukei d'zimra, preliminary blessings and psalms (Psalms 35:10), which he had missed reciting because of his lateness: "All my bones shall say, who is like You, God?" How then, Rav Simhah asked, could he come to pray before his bones were all awake?

Think of yoga: this form of exercise has an amazing ability to awaken the bones, lengthen your spine, ground your stance, and clear your mind, providing a deeper connection and understanding within yourself. It begins with setting an intention, a clear parallel to that of a blessing in a kosher diet. When I was younger, I didn't relate to the appeal of yoga, but as I matured, I grew to feel the benefits in my mind and see them on my body.

Similar to the benefit of connecting the physical act of eating with mindfulness as a method to help you overcome the barriers to weight loss, it is important to make a similar connection for fitness. In Judaism, there are daily prayers where we thank G–d for doing one of the scopes of performing yoga with the statement that He, "Straightens all who are bent." It helps to tap into our spiritual side by working on our physical one and provide more meaning to fitness so that we get it done.

Research shows benefits to yoga on our physical and emotional health. During yoga, your blood vessels relax and blood pressure reduces, while the blood flow to the heart increases. Research reported in the April 2015 *Journal of Diabetology & Metabolic Syndrome* followed 182 middle-aged Chinese adults who suffered from metabolic syndrome and practiced yoga for a year. Engaging in yoga not only lowered their blood pressure but also helped significantly slim them down.

Yoga also helps strengthen your mind. In a recent study of 133 older adults ages 53 to 96, the June 2015 issue of *Journal of Neuroscience Nursing* reported that those who engaged in 30 minutes of yoga twice a week for more than a month experienced improvement in their cognitive function. The focused breathing necessary in the poses of yoga maximizes oxygenation, and movement increases blood flow to brain and body. Participants not only had significant improvements in memory, but also fewer depressive symptoms. A new report presented at the Anxiety and Depression Association of America (ADAA) Conference in April 2015 connected yoga to lowering levels of cortisol, the stress hormone, especially in women at risk for mental health issues. One study of 52 women ages 25 to 45 who had mildly elevated anxiety, moderate depression, or high stress, performed Bikram yoga (a 90-minute heated form of Hatha yoga) twice a week and felt better (improved mood), looked better (lost weight), and had better control over their anxiety. In a pilot study from Brazil published in *Complementary Therapies in Clinical Practice* in May 2015, university students reported feeling better right after their yoga practice, especially about self-control, self-perception, well-being, body awareness, balance, mind-body, and reflexivity. Aside from obvious physical benefits we want to feel from yoga, the emotional ones are critical in encouraging you to stick with the diet and sustain the healthy habits after the 21 days.

## Daily Breakdown of Exercises

After you recite a morning meditation or my daily motivations at the start of each of the 21 days focusing on health and well-being, you can complete the fitness recommendation or other forms of activity listed in the suggested "Resources for Fitness" for 30 minutes to 1 hour at least four days per week. Throughout your day, grab at opportunities to keep walking (see "21 Ways to Keep Moving" below) so that you reach your recommended 10,000 steps. Be careful not to exercise for over 1 hour because the total calories and balance of meals and snacks would have to be modified. Remember, over-exercising is not useful on this plan and can potentially result in a lack of weight loss or weight gain if you overeat as a result.

## 21 Ways to Keep Moving

▶ Exercise regularly, make it a priority, but exercise smart with the forms I recommend: yoga, interval-based training, and walking. Increase the intensity and shorten the time to maximize fat burning.

▶ Aim for 30 to 60 minutes per day of yoga and/or interval based training, at least four days per week. Ideally, set up rest days so that they are not consecutive. Feel free to alter and combine different exercise modalities, but do not go over 1 hour because it will confuse your calorie needs and food timing.

▶ Our goal in this plan is to hit 10,000 steps each day. I recommend you purchase a simple pedometer to track your steps and log it in your Wellness Planner each day.

▶ Remember that working out on an empty stomach means you will end up burning fewer calories. Be sure to leave yourself 30 minutes before exercising after eating a snack and 60 minutes before exercising after eating a meal.

▶ Recovery eating after a workout is critical. Allow yourself to eat either a snack or a meal designated on the day's meal plan within 30 minutes after exercising. As you will read in chapter 4, if you do not eat at the indicated times, you will get hungrier later in the day.

▶ Similar signals in the brain trigger hunger and thirst. Pay attention to hydrating adequately with water before, during, and after your workout.

## Don't Plan Not to Succeed; It's Practice that Gets You There

It can be overwhelming to begin an exercise regimen, especially if you are not typically active. You may not feel comfortable going out into a group class or public gym because of how you look or if you feel exercise-inept. I cannot tell you how many people you see at these places that feel the same way. I know because many clients were walking into my office describing a degree of discomfort working out in public. If we realize each of us feels self-conscious on some level, we would get over it quickly and start exercising the right way as a fun, motivating, and uplifting activity.

Ultimately, you will only continue doing what you love. However, you won't know which type of fitness you like until you start somewhere and give the routine a fair shot by pursuing it long enough to catch on and improve. The exercises described for my diet are not only achievable at any level and able to be increased in intensity for those more advanced, but you can also perform them at your comfort level in your home or out in public and in a time crunch. The most important thing is that you start. You cannot achieve anything without a beginning. In the next chapter you will learn other strategic guidelines that will follow you throughout the 21 days. You already took the first step by choosing my diet, and you owe it to yourself to move in only one direction...forward.

See Appendix A (page 209) for suggested yoga poses and circuit training routines.

# CHAPTER 3

# Shopping for Soul Food

"As for you, take for yourself some of all food which is edible, and gather it to yourself; and it shall be for food for you and for them."

—GENESIS 6:21

Although keeping kosher means eating foods that are soul-friendly, my diet also incorporates foods that are friendly toward your mind and body. Unfortunately, not all kosher food products are inherently good for you. By combining my clean eating shopping list with my guide to purchasing kosher food, you will become David in the Goliath of supermarkets and win in the battle against the confusing world of packaged foods. In this chapter, I will teach you how to shop for the kosher foods that help facilitate weight loss.

Your focus on my plan is this: Choose from whole, less processed foods as often as possible to create your meals and snacks, while occasionally using packaged minimally processed products.

## Clean Eating Grocery List for Beginners

I love when I get the opportunity to fill up clients' pantries with whole foods or guide a group through the aisles of a supermarket and teach them how to shop for packaged products on my plan. The first section in a supermarket to buy is the perimeter, where they stock fresh fruits and vegetables. It's hard to go wrong when you stick with the strategy to buy whole foods that are more a product of G-d than a product of industry. But the anxiety grows as you enter the unchartered territory of the aisles that stock an overwhelming amount of packaged foods. I break down exactly what you need to look out for when you shop for foods on my plan with my Clean Eating Grocery List for Beginners. Although suggested products and brand names may require tweaks based on your local store availability, the overall ideas are a good place to start.

## What to Keep in Your Pantry

Following is a list of high-level ingredients to keep in your pantry during the 21-day plan and beyond:

- ▶ Lots of vegetables and plenty of fruit. Try to shop for produce at your local farmers' market and opt to purchase organic when possible. If budgeted, prioritize organic purchases of those identified by the Environmental Working Group (EWG) "Dirty Dozen" annual list (ewg.com) as having the most amount of pesticides used in conventional farming.

- ▶ Dairy products, including unsweetened yogurt and cheese. Purchase organic "whole" or "low-fat" varieties of milk products, which are less processed.

- ▶ 100 percent whole-grains. Ideally, buy brands of grains, such as bread, with a minimal amount of ingredients and ones that you can pronounce. For an improved glycemic response on blood sugar and better gastrointestinal tolerance, purchase sprouted whole grain varieties and sourdough bread.

- ▶ Fish. Wild caught is optimal over farm-raised. Remember: shellfish are not kosher and only fish with fins and scales are deemed kosher (see more in the "How to Shop for Kosher Foods" section on page 39).

- ▶ Beef, chicken, and turkey. Ideally, purchase local grass-fed or pasture-raised animal products. Red meat will be provided as an option 1 to 2 times per week and should be Glatt kosher ("glatt" means "smooth" in Yiddish and refers to the lack of adhesions on the lungs of an animal).

- ▶ Beverages limited to water, coffee, tea, and non-dairy milk. All natural juices are not included in the plan during the 21 days due to the high sugar content.

## KITCHEN EQUIPMENT

Aside from the basic kitchen equipment including pots and pans, here are some items that you may not have but are needed to create recipes on the plan:

- A strong blender such as Ninja or Vitamix—This isn't mandatory, but it improves texture and ease of making a lot of the recipes.
- Food processor—You may not need this if you have a good blender.
- Cast iron skillet
- Spiralizer—You can opt to use a vegetable grater instead or simply chop the vegetable.
- Grill pan or grill

▶ Other approved snacks include dried fruit with no added sugar or preservatives, seeds and nuts, along with fresh popcorn made with organic kernels.

▶ All natural sweeteners including honey, 100 percent maple syrup, and fruit juice concentrates are acceptable in moderation during maintenance. On our 21-day plan, they will be profoundly limited and used only in some calculated marinade recipes along with natural non-calorie sweeteners such as pure stevia and monk fruit extract.

## A Deep Dive into Each Shopping Category

### Clean Dairy and Non-Dairy Options

I do not eliminate any macronutrient on the plan if it provides an advantage for our health. However, I do not require consumption of any one food group if someone does not tolerate it. Although dairy is somewhat controversial in wellness circles, it is proven beneficial to one's health.[15] If you are lactose intolerant, allergic, or discover an intolerance to dairy while following the plan, you can swap it for another protein source (see the Meal Exchange List on page 64).

The typical rule-of-thumb is to purchase full-fat or low-fat varieties of dairy. Believe it or not, science agrees that consuming full-fat dairy did not significantly cause weight gain.[16] Because dairy is a source of saturated fat, may pose an intolerance to many if over-consumed, and can contribute to weight gain due to its high sodium and calorie content in cheese, for example, it is rotated among the other macronutrients during the 21 days and not consumed daily. While I favor dairy as a protein, calcium, and vitamin D source along with potassium and other nutrients, we can get these nutrients adequately from eating a variety of whole foods including salmon, almonds, legumes, and vegetable.

▶ **Cow's milk**—Any form of legal milk has some processing, which is why my plan focuses on "less-processed" as opposed to "non-processed" foods. Homogenization, for example, is a form of processing dairy to keep the milk homogenized and not separated. The next best thing to milking a cow yourself is to purchase organic full-fat milk. You can opt to buy low-fat dairy products, but the reduction in fat is accompanied by a higher level of processing and move further from the natural whole food source. Ideally, purchase organic, grass-fed varieties of milk when available.

▶ **Yogurt**—Greek yogurt is ideal because of its high source of protein. The plain flavor is the best choice since it is free of artificial sweeteners and added sugars. Keep an open mind if it is your first time trying a non-flavored yogurt. My recipes include mixing the plain yogurt with flavorful foods, such as fruit and granola, to make it taste like an entirely new dish. You can also purchase skyr plain yogurt, such as Siggi's, which has less natural sugar, no added sugar, and is high in protein.

If you opt for non-dairy alternatives to yogurt, such as coconut milk and almond milk, then purchase unsweetened varieties.

▶ **Cheese**—Overall, cheese promotes temptation to overeat the appropriate portion. Most kosher natural cheeses are okay to consume, but moderately, because of their high saturated fat content and high sodium level. You can save cost by shredding your cheese, which has the added benefit of avoiding anti-caking agents sometimes used on pre-shredded cheese. Full or low-fat cottage cheese is also approved.

▶ **Unsweetened Almond Milk**—If you can't make your own, look for a brand of almond milk without additives such as carrageenan.

There are other varieties of unsweetened non-dairy milk including unsweetened rice, cashew, hemp, and coconut milk that can be used as alternatives. While on the 21-day plan, be sure to use the milk and yogurt alternatives recommended because of the calculated nutrient and calorie distribution. If you are allergic to dairy, then you can substitute another non-dairy option from the Meal Exchange List.

### Bottom Line Clean Dairy Sources

▶ Plain yogurt; Milk; Cheese; Unsweetened non-dairy milk (free of carrageenan and other preservatives); Greek yogurt; Cottage cheese; Cheese (goat, Parmesan, ricotta, feta)

▶ Clean Non-Dairy Alternatives: Unsweetened plain almond, cashew, hemp, rice and coconut milk (made without additives such as carrageenan).

## Clean Protein Options

Quality protein plays a critical role in facilitating weight loss and enhancing meal satisfaction. You may consume grass-fed meats such as chicken breast and chicken thigh, Glatt kosher sirloin, and lean ground beef, which are acceptable at designated times on my plan. Even though wellness advocates either hate or love red meat, research consistently shows that there is a benefit to limiting red meat for your overall health.[17] I offer red meat as a protein option on my meal plan on the Sabbath (Friday night and Saturday meals), which is the optimal time to eat something different and special if a person can afford the expense, according to the Rambam in his book, Mishnah Torah, chapter 5. Meat is also a unique iron source and contains coveted vitamin B$_{12}$ found in animal proteins. Luckily for us, when following a kosher diet, Glatt kosher also ensures that you are eating humanely slaughtered beef. One type of meat not recommended on the plan, ironically, is the modern cultural kosher food, deli. When you eat clean, it means avoiding heavily processed meats such as bologna, salami, and hot dogs often filled with nitrates, sodium, preservatives, and artificial coloring.

Fish are a lean protein source that contains different anti-inflammatory heart-healthy omega-3 fats, EPA, and DHA, to varying degrees.

Choose kosher sustainably sourced fish when possible by checking out seafoodwatch.org. Even though most fish high in mercury are non-kosher, my meal plan rotates different types of fish to help keep your intake of mercury low.

Eggs are another underestimated super-protein source, including the nutrient-rich yolk that is unfairly scandalized. In the 2015 Healthy Guidelines for Americans, eggs were no longer identified as a food of concern. It turned out that it is the saturated fat content in the diet as a whole that breeds an increased risk of heart disease, not the poor egg yolk alone. Ideally, choose pasture-raised eggs and if they are not available or out of your price range, opt for organic varieties with omega-3 fats. Nuts, seeds, unprocessed soy, and beans can count toward plant-based proteins. Look out for sodium-free varieties while shopping and check the portion size designated on my meal plan before eating.

### Bottom Line Clean Protein Sources

▶ Single-ingredient meats include grass-fed chicken breast, chicken legs, ground beef, cuts of red meat, and turkey. All red meat should be Glatt kosher.

▶ Fish—choose sustainable kosher options, such as wild salmon and Pacific cod. Check seafoodwatch.org for a list of the best choices.

▶ Eggs—pasture-raised, ideally, or organic with omega-3 varieties.

▶ Raw nuts and seeds—including almonds, cashews, hazelnuts, walnuts, hemp, sunflower, sesame, pumpkin, chia, and flaxseed.

▶ Unflavored natural nut butter (no added sugar).

▶ Dried beans and canned beans including lentils, black beans, chickpeas (garbanzo beans), and kidney beans, ideally no sodium and packed in BPA-free cans.

▶ Unprocessed soy products—organic tofu, organic tempeh, edamame.

## Clean Produce

Finally, a category where you can unleash your frenzy while clean kosher food shopping. I encourage you to embrace "the more, the merrier" attitude when it comes to filling your plate with a wide variety of non-starchy veggies when indicated on my kosher girl's diet (see the Meal Exchange List on page 64). Vegetables are the foundation of your meals because they are low in calories and packed with vitamins, minerals, water, and fiber. Although you should not mindlessly munch on any food, vegetables can be considered "free foods" and eaten only in conjunction with any meal or snack.

Because of the attention to the distribution of a lot of veggies on your plate, they become the food that fills you up the most during a meal. It's the balance of a dish that provides a different feeling of fullness than skewing your dish more heavily toward carbohydrates. Frozen vegetables are allowed and can sometimes be more budget-friendly, quicker to prepare, and nutrient rich. Other vegetables, such as potatoes and winter squash, are starchy. Starchy vegetables are counted toward a carbohydrate on my diet and are therefore not considered unlimited (see the Meal Exchange List).

Fresh fruit is typically a clean and kosher choice. Fruits are placed strategically throughout the day in the meal plan for reasons similar to eating vegetables. Because they contain natural sugars, you can eat fruit in the specified quantity and timing dictated by the meal plan and are not considered "free." Be wary of added sugars in canned or dried fruits because they provide empty calories, can easily be overeaten, and trigger cravings.

I encourage you to be mindful of your food budget when it comes down to choosing whether to buy organic or conventional produce. As a general rule of thumb, attempt to purchase organic fruits and vegetables that have thin skin such as peaches, nectarines, and all berries, while buying conventional produce that has thicker skin like bananas and oranges. Check out the EWG annual list of "The Dirty Dozen" to keep track of the worst pesticide-laden produce and the "Clean 15" for the ideal produce to purchase conventionally.

### Fruit Juice

Fruit juice should be avoided on the 21-day plan but can be used in limited amounts in the maintenance phase. Keep in mind that some juices can contain almost 30 grams of sugar per 8-ounce serving. Fruit juices are missing beneficial fiber found in whole fruits, even if it is 100 percent pure. You are also more likely to guzzle additional calories by drinking juice rather than eating a whole fruit, spurring cravings for more sweets, which is in large part a reason to avoid juices during the 21 days.

### Dried Fruit

Dried fruit can come in handy for that nagging sweet tooth in a multitude of helpful ways on my 21-day plan, including the optional after dinner snack. When buying dried fruit, steer clear of any with added sweeteners or preservatives such as sulfur dioxide. You want to look for "raw" or "natural" fruit that with "no added sugar" and make sure to portion-control the fruit before eating it.

### Bottom Line Clean Produce Options

▶ Purchase organic vegetables and fruits on "The Dirty Dozen" list (ewg.org), but otherwise, conventional produce is acceptable. Additive-free frozen fruits and vegetables are permitted.

▶ Dried fruit with no added sugar can be used on a limited basis.

## Whole Grains

Nutritious and fiber-rich whole grains such as brown rice, quinoa, barley, oats, farro, and millet are naturally both clean and kosher. When it comes to other whole grain products, such as bread and pasta, look for 100 percent varieties and ingredients that list whole-wheat flour first and contain no added sugar. Whole grains are a once-a-day carbohydrate option on my kosher girl's diet. Interestingly, popcorn also counts as a carb, but in the form of a starchy vegetable. I recommended you buy the corn kernels and pop them on the stove or in an air popper for a clean snack without the additives, buttery calories, and toxins found in microwave bags of popcorn.

### Bottom Line Clean Whole-Grain Sources

▶ Single-ingredient grains, such as farro, millet, oats, barley, quinoa, brown rice, and so forth

▶ 100 percent whole-wheat, brown rice, or quinoa pasta

▶ Sprouted whole-grain bread and English muffins (no added sugar)

## A NOTE ON CANNED FOODS

There is debate as to whether or not canned items are a clean ingredient due to the Bisphenol-A (BPA) in the lining of the can. Today, there are BPA-free cans on the market, such as Eden foods. If you have the budget and the availability, it would be a better choice to purchase BPA-free cans that are certified kosher.

If you decide to buy foods like beans, tomato sauce, or tomato paste in a can you should read the ingredients. You are looking to buy cans with no added sugar, which include ingredients labeled as sugar, evaporated cane juice, dextrose, fructose, corn syrup, or high fructose corn syrup. Also, opt for no- or low-sodium canned goods when available and rinse the food in water to get rid of the excess salt by 35 percent. When using a canned food already prepared with sodium, try not to add additional salt to the recipe.

- ▶ Popcorn
- ▶ Sourdough whole grain breads
- ▶ Whole wheat breadcrumbs (or Panko), gluten-free flours such as coconut, garbanzo, almond, quinoa, and brown rice (no white rice flours)

### Sauces

Innocently, you may snag canned or jarred sauce or salsa from the store shelves thinking they are all equivalent products. Unfortunately, there are many hidden ingredients and artificial food colorings blatant among brands. Make sure the ingredient list does not contain added sugars, additives, or artificial colors, especially in products like mustard, pickles, and ketchup.

### Seasonings

Purchasing spices and herbs are not as clear-cut as it seems. It is best to prepare fresh garlic, ginger, and spice combinations yourself and store them in the refrigerator or freezer in an ice cube tray for easy use. Although we welcome a shortcut among our busy schedules, I do not recommend items such as pre-chopped garlic, which contains superfluous sulfur dioxide to preserve freshness and may include added salt and sugar.

It is also important to keep an eye out for flavorings, such as vanilla, to ensure you are not purchasing an imitation, only the pure form with no added chemicals or sugars. If you have the budget, buy a vanilla pod to scrape for vanilla, which also adds a burst of flavor.

### Bottom Line Clean Seasonings and Spices

▶ **Spices:** Any herbs you buy should come in bulk or a bottle. Do not purchase seasoning packets. Buy singular herbs such as basil, parsley, and thyme (unless otherwise noted on the Shopping List). Opt for garlic and onion powder without salt.

▶ **Salt:** Although salt is an ingredient in most recipes, you should be mindful of added salt in the diet as it relates to your weight. Getting a good quality salt, such as sea salt, is important but kosher salt and table salt are also present in some recipes and moderated.

▶ **Other Approved Condiments:** Hot sauce; vinegar (red wine vinegar, balsamic, apple cider, and so forth); Dijon mustard; reduced-sodium soy sauce, and Tamari (see the Unlimited section in part 3)

## Clean Fats

### Oils, Margarine, and Spreadable Butters

It will be difficult to find what we refer to as "*pareve*" (see the next section) or non-dairy, spreadable butter that is not highly processed. Your best bet is to go with a portioned amount of unrefined coconut oil when you need a spreadable semi-solid option on my plan for certain recipe consistencies and high heat cooking. Although it's a clean and kosher plant-based ingredient, a recent study reconfirmed that the saturated fat content in coconut oil still poses a problem for heart health and should be used moderately.[18] Cheaper oils and chemically hardened vegetable oils create the processed form of spreadable oil. These contain trans-fat, the bad inflammatory fat that we want to avoid for weight loss and better health.

Butter—although butter made headlines again after a published study in 2016 concluded butter isn't the enemy ingredient for your health, most cardiologists rebuffed the findings, citing consistent research showing to limit any form of saturated fat for heart health.[19] In reality, it is hard to find a less processed organic, certified kosher butter. On my 21-day meal plan, we will incorporate liquid vegetable oils and unrefined coconut oil, as directed.

### Bottom Line Clean Fat Sources

▶ Extra-virgin olive oil, sesame oil, coconut oil, avocado oil, walnut oil

## Sweeteners

One goal during the 21 days is to decrease your sweet tooth. I work with a delicate balance between restricting sweets altogether, which may result in a binge of cookies as soon as you see them in front of you, and over-loading on too many processed sweets, which includes 100-calorie snack packs of cookies and dietetic muffins. My goal is to sensitize your palette to become satisfied after eating foods with natural sweetness and at times fewer amounts of packaged foods with minimal added natural sweeteners to keep your cravings at bay. A manufacturer can create a heavily processed sugar alternative as a form of agave, stevia, and commercially-produced honey, but you can find options with more "clean" ingredients. My first choice would be pure stevia or monk fruit extract. Other sweeteners that are less processed and limited during the 21 days are raw Manuka honey, pure maple syrup, and unsulfured molasses.

### Bottom Line Clean Sweeteners

The plan is designed to limit added sugar intake as much as possible. However, when you want your weekly clean treat (discussed in part 3) or create a designated recipe on my kosher girl's diet, the following sweeteners approved include: Date sugar, raw honey, pure maple syrup, Sucanat, unsulfured molasses, pure stevia, monk fruit extract, agave syrup, agave nectar, coconut sugar

## A LETTER FROM DEBBIE

Debbie, age 30 and mom of four, found me through social media (@beth_warren Instagram account) all the way from Zurich, Switzerland. We interacted via Skype throughout her journey on my 21-day diet. Debbie had to overcome many challenges to be successful on the plan, including limited access both to fresh and packaged kosher foods. She adapted the meal plan to fit her lifestyle beautifully and often had to make ingredients, such as almond milk, from scratch. Her determination and effort pushed her through to completion of the 21 days successfully. Here is an email she wrote me one year later:

*It has now been a year since your kosher cleanse and hakol letova (Hebrew for everything's for the best) since I can now give you a feedback after one year that's even more impactful.*

*First of all, I cannot thank you enough for exposing me to clean eating and feeling great. Despite the hard work in making everything from scratch here in Switzerland, I learned that if you are organized and prepared nothing is impossible, just a lot of work, but worth it. I have made the quinoa crust pizza so many times, I make double and freeze it. My kids love it too. You truly helped change not only me, but my family as well through my efforts to cook and eat clean, kosher foods.*

*Since I got your first book I use it as my guideline, how many nuts as snacks, etc...and keep recommending it to so many Jewish people.*

*Looking for healthy kosher products in the stores and market in Zurich has become my hobby. I get asked by Jewish ladies here what can they replace things with to make it healthier and kosher. I have regular contact with the local rabbi trying to get cheaper and kosher alternatives, you've turned me into an advocator for better health for my entire community! I enjoy it and love helping others. So the consequences are that I am currently doing a nutrition course online and looking into a coaching one too after summer.... I am far from being a certified nutritionist as these are just small courses but I do it more for my knowledge and fun.*

*Thanks to you I have learned a lot and most importantly that by eating clean not only do you lose weight but feel better altogether.*

*I have to admit that I also enjoy the good food in life and also cheat here and there and I can't skip my coffee in the morning, but I try to have a balance, and it works for me. You taught me not to feel guilty about what I truly need, and for that, I feel motivated to eat better the rest of the time.*

*During the three weeks cleanse last year, I felt a difference on my skin, cycle (my period had less clotting and wasn't as heavy) and felt more energetic.*

*Now that Passover is done, I am starting the cleansing challenge again and taking your book and last year's notes as a guideline.*
*Thank you for your inspiration and motivation.*
*Shabbat Shalom,*
*Debbie*

## Beverages

When you go shopping, try to choose organic fair-trade coffee and teas. While water is the ideal beverage, you can also drink seltzers that do not contain non-calorie sweeteners or sugars. You will read more about how to fit drinks including tea, coffee, and red wine into my diet in chapter 4.

## Miscellaneous Approved Clean Ingredients

- ▸ Low-sodium chicken or vegetable broth
- ▸ Cacao nibs
- ▸ Dark chocolate, at least 70 percent cacao
- ▸ Unsweetened shredded coconut
- ▸ Unsweetened cocoa powder

# How to Shop for Kosher Food Products

The laws of Kashrus include a comprehensive "rulebook" of permitted and forbidden foods. This section will take you through the relevant aspects of kosher dietary law you will encounter while shopping.

## Understanding the Kosher Market

More than 80 percent of the products offered by the food industry contain pre-processed ingredients that need to have kosher supervision. About three-quarters of packaged foods in the United States are certified kosher and bear a *hechsher* (Hebrew for "kosher approval") symbol. Although looking for a *hechsher* adds another layer on top of what you already need to consider while grocery shopping for clean foods, it is sure to keep you intensely focused on food labels and packaging so that you make the right choice for your weight loss goals. Clean ingredients are not guaranteed to be inherent within kosher food products, but you will become an expert at shopping for goods that will help you lose weight by combining designated kosher rules with my clean eating shopping guidelines.

You won't be the only person looking to purchase kosher food at the supermarket, regardless of religion. Not only Jewish people buy kosher food. Some consumers prefer kosher foods because it is perceived to be safer or more wholesome. A large number of shoppers in the industry include people seeking kosher food for health reasons. Shoppers may be lactose-intolerant consumers who buy pareve products (see the following), which contain neither meat nor dairy ingredients, along with vegans, vegetarians, and people with food allergies who favor kosher foods because the industry's labeling practices are considered to be more rigorous. Consumers also view kosher meat as healthier than typical non-kosher meat because of the strict rules regarding the slaughter and inspection of animals.

Here are three categories of kosher foods that you should know about on my plan: dairy, meat, and pareve. Pareve foods are neutral foods such as bread, fruits, and vegetables that have neither had contact with milk or meat, nor are they prepared with dairy or meat. Pareve foods are mostly kosher unless they are combined or made with dairy or meat foods.

## How to Distinguish Kosher Food Products

It will help to familiarize yourself with *hechsher* symbols, which are specialized certifications that indicate kosher food preparation and packaging, before going shopping. Look online for a list of *hechsher* symbols printed on kosher food packages in various nations.[20] A simple capital "K" does not necessarily mean a rabbi supervised food preparation, but some reliable *hechsher* symbols incorporate a K. Similarly, an "R" in a circle, like this ®, is a registered trademark, and it does not indicate kosher foods.

## What Foods Need a Hechsher

To buy strictly kosher food products on my program, you should know which types need a kosher symbol. Look for the *hechsher* on all breakfast cereals, cheeses, baked goods, sauces, pasta, canned fish, condiments, and ground spices. Check that all prepared foods had rabbinic supervision during the process and bore a kosher symbol as well.

Keep in mind that some products do not require kosher certification. Without mixing a product that grew from the earth with any oils or other products most likely makes it kosher. These items include raw nuts, flour, wheat, oats, vegetables, fruits, popcorn kernels, soybeans, rice, spices, unflavored teas, and coffee.

Even though it is recommended to make the meals on the plan from scratch, at times you may need to buy certain prepared foods from commercial establishments. Aside from making sure these places use whole food ingredients on the plan, it is also important to go to butchers, restaurants, and other supervised facilities by rabbis or a *"mashgiach."* Many people assume this means the rabbi blesses the food, but it is a lot more involved than that. A rabbi will oversee the process of preparation to ensure the use of only kosher ingredients and cooking equipment.

## How to Buy Kosher Products

### Meats and Fish

If you shop for meats and poultry in a supermarket, buy whole kosher chickens with a *plumba* attached, which is a small metal tag with a *hechsher*. A *plumba* is appended to the bag if a chicken is cut up. Buy kosher meats only from the front quarters of the animal. Be sure prepared meat had rabbinic supervision by a butcher deemed reliable in kosher practice. On the plan, it is recommended you also consume organic grass-fed kosher chicken.

When it comes to buying fish, purchase the types that have fins and scales because those that do not are non-kosher. Fish must have scales that can be removed with a knife or by hand without ripping the underlying skin. On my diet, it is recommended you buy wild-caught varieties.

### Dairy

Hard cheeses need kosher certification because of the rennet used, which can sometimes come from calves' stomachs. Milk, butter, and cream are considered kosher.

*Eggs*

The eggs of kosher birds are fit to eat as long as they do not contain blood. Therefore, you need to individually examine all eggs, especially the organic variety recommended on my plan that tends to have more blood.

*Fruits, Vegetables, Cereals*

All products that grow in the soil or on plants, bushes, or trees are kosher. However, all insects and animals that have many legs or very short legs are not kosher. Consequently, check vegetables, fruits, and other products infested with insects and remove the bugs. Carefully inspect plants prone to insect infestation (e.g., cauliflower).

*Kosher Wine*

While on my diet, I take into account the red wine needed to make the blessing of Kiddish during the Sabbath. The wine has strict kosher laws associated with its production, packaging, and handling, and therefore must bear a kosher symbol.

## DECIPHERING FOOD LABELS

Food labels are often read incorrectly. It may help to think of the "JUST" rule when looking at a package's ingredients. For example, peanut butter should technically JUST have peanuts as the ingredient and tomato sauce should JUST have tomatoes. Therefore, your goal when choosing the cleanest product is to narrow down ingredients to be as close to "JUST" the ingredients necessary to make the product. You can also ask yourself the question, "Why am I buying the product? For what food group category?" For example:

- **Carbohydrates:** Most carbohydrates per serving provide about the same or within a range of 20 to 30 calories from each other per serving. If you were to look only at the calories of the product, it will not tell you enough of what you need to know about choosing a food product as a source of carbohydrate. Therefore, first checkout the grams of carbs, fiber, and sugar to help you make the best choice for the food group.
- **Added sugars:** See the sidebar "What to Avoid" on page 41 to identify the sneaky names for added sugars in a product. The goal is to limit

sources of added sugar as much as possible. If you can opt to choose a product with 0 to 2 types of sugar over one with 5 to 6, obviously choose the one with less sources of natural sugar, such as brown rice syrup, and no processed sugar such as high fructose corn syrup.

- **Fiber content:** When purchasing foods in the carbohydrate category, it is important to choose an option with at least 2 to 3 grams or more of natural, not fortified, fiber or over 5 grams when it comes to cereal.

- **Fats:** All fats are not created equal. Calories aside, try taking a deeper dive into what types of fats are in the product. The goal is to eat more of anti-inflammatory monounsaturated and polyunsaturated fats, less pro-inflammatory saturated fat, and no trans fat (which includes any product with the words "partially hydrogenated" in the food label, even if it is listed as "0 grams trans fat").

- **Protein:** The amount of protein is not the deciding factor in whether or not to purchase a quality packaged products, mostly because it is in most foods. For example, if a cereal such as Special K adds protein, but you are counting the cereal as a carbohydrate, then the protein content is less relevant. Therefore, you would use the methods described in how to choose a quality carbohydrate food product to make your decision on a healthy cereal and less regard to the fact that the product added protein.

## How to Shop for Clean Kosher Foods on a Budget

Let's face it, one of the most common obstacles in the way of buying healthy foods is the cost. Here are some ways to save money while on the plan:

1. Avoid "superfoods." It's always more interesting to try out foods like maca powder if the budget allows, but you can eat a wholesome diet without these ingredients in the recipes.

2. Cut down on packaged and pre-made. Convenience costs money, so don't plan on buying packaged and pre-made food items already prepared. My plan recommends you make and shop one day per week. Stick to the schedule, and it will be easier to fit the plan into your busy life.

3. Eat leftovers. While following the meal plan, I help you utilize each ingredient to its maximum over the course of the 21 days. I also carry over leftovers into the following days' meals or recommend you freeze individual items to be used at a later time on the plan. These strategies help minimize food and money waste.

4. Know when to skip organic. We can't all afford only organic products, and it is not as critical if it makes healthy food choices harder to maintain.

5. Shop online. These days it is sometimes less expensive and more convenient to shop for foods online than in-store.

6. Buy in-season produce. You can save money and ensure maximum nutrition by opting to buy seasonal produce. During the other months, try buying frozen, which is also cost-effective.

7. Buy in bulk. Ingredients including nuts and seeds or flours that can be expensive, including almond flour, can be purchased in bulk if it saves cost.

8. Scan store brands. Simply because store brands may be cheaper, does not mean they have less nutrition than brand names. Compare price tags and purchase the more affordable option when all other ingredients are equal.

9. Go shopping with your meal plan and a shopping list to follow. By sticking to the ingredient list provided for each week, you will be less likely to overspend on other items.

10. Scope out other possible shopping venues. You may need to shop in a smaller specialty store if you are new to purchasing clean and kosher foods when you start the plan, but once you feel comfortable with the products you can start to buy in places with the best prices. Although time-consuming at first, it is a good idea to scope out local stores to figure out what products are the best prices in various locations.

11. Watch for sales. Be sure to check out a store's weekly circular for sales and browse online and in print publications for coupons.

**See Appendix B (page 223) for the full Weekly Shopping List.**

## WHAT TO AVOID

Products with the following ingredients are going to be eliminated while following the 21-day plan both for kosher and health reasons. You can identify them by browsing the ingredient list on the actual food label on the side or back of the package. Be careful about misleading advertising at the front of the label of food packages; it's a novice mistake. Follow this list as an example, but the rule of thumb is to keep out foods with ingredients we cannot pronounce, contain more ingredients than are needed, and include inherently non-kosher ingredients:

- No refined grains such as white flour or white rice (items containing wheat must say whole wheat, not just "wheat"). Ideally, grains will be sprouted or fermented.
- No refined sweeteners such as sugar, any form of corn syrup, cane juice, or artificial sweeteners such as Equal, Sweet n' Low, or Splenda.
- Products with added preservatives and chemicals such as BHA and BHT, carrageenan, maltodextrin, disodium inosinate, disodium guanylate, modified cornstarch, and artificial food coloring (such as "FD&C" with any number following)
- Products with multiple sources of added sugar, which include ingredients labeled sugar, evaporated cane juice, dextrose, fructose, corn syrup, or high fructose corn syrup, as much as possible
- Monosodium glutamate
- Soybean oil
- Processed meats AKA "deli"
- Textured soy protein concentrate including soy protein isolate

# Part Two
# GET (MIND) SET

*"It is better to know well*
*than to know much."*
—MISHLE YEHOSHUA

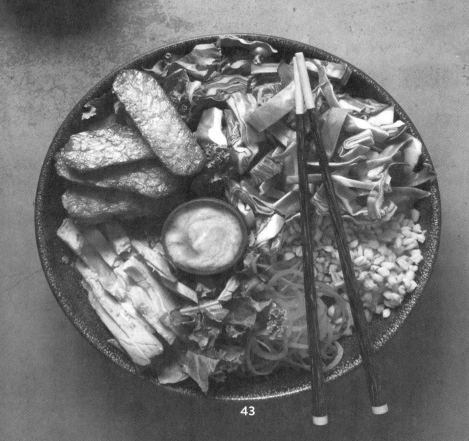

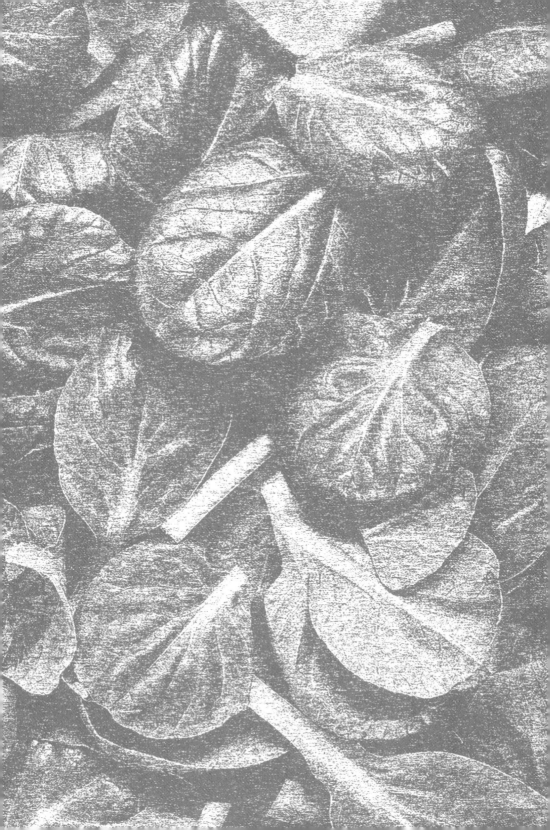

# CHAPTER 4

# Timing Is Everything

*"If you understand the why and wherefore of what you learn, you do not forget it quickly."*

—TALMUD YERUSHALMI, BERAKOT 5:1

My pet peeve is when people follow a diet without understanding its strategy. Often a plan lacks consistency, such as forbidding carbohydrates yet allowing a starchy sweet potato, or indicating fruits as unlimited even though they contain calories and sugar that should factor into a weight loss plan. The consequences of not knowing the methodology make it unlikely to sustain weight loss. The odds are that in life you will face unknown circumstances that will throw your diet off-kilter, such as a birthday party, social gathering, or trip to a new grocery store. In the heat of the moment, you will not know how to adapt the diet to real-world scenarios and "fall off." During the 21 days of my diet, I provide you with daily meals, snacks, and recipes you need to follow to lose weight. However, in this chapter, I will unveil the building blocks of my diet so you can make it through unexpected times successfully during the plan and beyond.

The goal is to strictly follow the actual meal plans and recipes I dictate in part 3. The plan as outlined is what guarantees the weight loss and other results. However, it is important to have the practical knowledge of how to perform the diet on your terms with substitutions in the event you are in an unexpected situation and can be successful long-term.

## The Rules of Engagement on My Kosher Girl's Diet

▶ Weigh yourself one time per week, not daily. Weighing yourself too often messes with your mood and motivation while you're on the plan.

▶ Limit added sugars. Because one goal is to decrease your sweet tooth, we are limiting added sugars and enhancing satisfaction from natural sweeteners in whole foods and less processed packaged products.

▶ Time your meals and snacks. Placing yourself on an eating schedule keeps your insulin and blood sugar levels in sync. The goal is to experience small peaks and valleys of insulin release, not sharp spikes and dips, which helps balance your hunger/fullness levels and prevent overeating, especially at night.

▶ Combine food choices. The recommended food combinations help ensure you feel both full and satisfied.

▶ Follow the treat per week rule. Both kosher and scientifically proven concepts, the practice keeps your emotional state uplifted and reinforces a healthy relationship with all types of food.

▶ Drink up on more fluids. By rotating various forms of liquid, you will keep hydrated on a diet, which not only affects weight in and of itself but also helps ward off inaccurate feelings of hunger.

▶ Abide by relevant kosher laws. It is a helpful strategy to use appropriate kosher legislation to enhance compliance on a diet.

By understanding the rules, you will be able to practically apply the plan to real life scenarios resulting in short-term weight loss and the knowledge of how to maintain the results.

## Timing Is Everything

Whip out those smartphones and get your calendar reminders ready. Eating at scheduled times is non-negotiable on my diet. A 2013 study in the *International Journal of Obesity*, titled "Timing of Food Intake Predicts Weight Loss Effectiveness," agreed that timing of eating is essential for weight loss in its conclusion stating, *"Eating late may influence the success of weight-loss therapy. Novel therapeutic strategies should incorporate not only the caloric intake and macronutrient distribution, as is classically done, but also the timing of food."*[21]

The missing piece of the hunger puzzle is the knowledge of what, when, and how much to eat so that you stoke your body's metabolizing engine 24/7. It's the peaks and dips in energy levels triggered by inconsistent eating habits that send cravings into overdrive and cause weight gain. On my diet, you will put yourself on an eating schedule as an added strategy to help you lose weight. The objective is not to feel force-fed, but to reset hunger and satiety cues so that you eat optimally for boosting metabolism and burning fat. The ultimate goal is to eat when you start to feel hungry and to stop eating when you are satisfied, ideally not when full and not when stuffed. Before starting my plan, your hunger-satiety cues are skewed or ignored. Most likely, you were previously eating when you were starving and stopping when you were either full or stuffed. At worst, you were the type of person that "wasn't hungry all day" and later overate throughout the evening and into the night. Simply put, you were eating to survive or "let-go", not to nourish your body.

At times, people incorrectly assume eating during the day will cause overeating because they opened up their appetite. Because of the warped rationale, they will ignore hunger pangs because they associate them with losing more weight. In reality, the opposite effect could be happening. These are the dieters who remark, "I'm good all day. I don't eat, but I'm gaining weight!" Here's what is happening: by skipping meals and snacks, you are putting your body into "starvation" mode. This storage state slows down metabolism, stores calories, and stops burning fat efficiently. If you experience weight loss during starvation mode, it is likely loss of muscle because your body is breaking it down to survive. Eating about every 2 to 4 hours throughout the day on my plan does not mean you are piling up calories to create more fat. On the contrary, you are shifting your metabolism into fat burning gear necessary for steady weight loss.

On the other hand, feeling the opposite end of the appetite spectrum, starving, is not optimal for weight loss either. When the body becomes overly hungry, blood sugar and insulin drops, causing powerful carbohydrate cravings, the likelihood of overeating at your next meal or snack, and "catch up" eating throughout the day, evening, and night. You know you reached a point of no return when it comes to satisfying your appetite once you feel an endless pit deep inside your stomach that cannot be filled no matter what foods you eat. Starving is the worst enemy to a sustainable diet because inevitably your food intake will spiral out of control.

Happily, starving is a feeling you will not experience on my diet. One consistent feedback I receive is the physical state of satisfaction from foods and recipes on the plan. In the beginning, you may think you are hungry; however, the feeling is not entirely truthful. It is amazing how your digestive system adapts when you keep consistent on the times of eating and balance of foods. You will not only become full and satisfied, but experience an added benefit of weight loss as well. Working on molding your hunger and fullness patterns is critical to help avoid weight gain from the ripple effect of not eating all day and subsequently overeating at night.

Technically, there is a degree of flexibility regarding eating times. You can swap the assigned daily meals and snacks as long as you consume either option in the allotted time slot. Let's say, for example, you are driving carpool for your kids or busy at work and cannot eat a full meal but you can manage a quick snack; you can swap the options. Your eating schedule may also change based on when you wake up. Although I advise starting calories early in the morning, as the *International Journal of Obesity* study found to be beneficial, it won't make or break your weight loss if you opt to start your day at 10:00 AM once in a while. During these times, eat at as soon as you wake up and subsequently adjust the meals and snacks accordingly to be at least two hours apart to end by 7 to 9 p.m. Remember that one goal of my diet is to make the plan as practical as possible while maintaining the essential framework that promotes weight loss.

## Bottom Line on Time

Eating should begin within one hour after waking up to switch your body into fat burning mode and subsequently spread out over 2-4 hours during the day. While there is no clear indicator of the best time to stop eating at night, generally speaking, the later it gets, the less likely you are eating out of hunger and more out of boredom, stress, or similar feelings.[22] If you are up too late or it reaches four hours after you previously ate at night, you may start to feel hungry again if you are forcing your body to stay awake because food provides energy; however, you should be listening to sleep cues and get some shut-eye instead of eating.

## Importance of Sleep

Sleep is critical for weight loss. It may be shocking, but if a client's patterns are off, my goal is to work out how to fix the sleep issue as much as the food one. Without quality sleep, cortisol, the stress hormone that puts your body in storage mode, increases. A lack of sleep leaves you craving more carbohydrates and likely to eat more calories in the latter part of the day.[23] A recent study found that participants ate significantly more calories from sugary carbohydrates after five and a half hours of slumber than they did after eight and a half hours. Experts aren't clear on why, but some think that less sleep causes ghrelin, the appetite-stimulating hormone, to spike.

Both modern science and multiple ancient Jewish sources including Maimonides agree that the goal is to get 6 to 8 hours of uninterrupted sleep. As a mom of five little ones, I know quality sleep is as close to a dream as we can expect to experience, but it is the ideal goal. If circumstances prevent you from getting sleep, it helps to flag those symptoms as they come up during the day. Keeping the commitment to any diet can be more difficult with the sleepless anchor weighing you down, but it is possible to achieve your goals as long as you are aware of its consequences and work harder to push through them.

The best time to sleep may seem obvious—during the night. One reason why, however, may not be as apparent. Your metabolism functions in a pattern regardless of whether or not you are awake or asleep. Therefore, if you keep awake at night, you should stick to eating your calories during the day. It is more challenging helping people who work night shifts lose weight. The brain has a master biological clock affected by light, which tells "peripheral" clocks in the muscles and organs the time of day. Because of these clocks, many of the metabolic processes that take place inside us operate at different rates over the course of a 24-hour period.

Dr. Freuman, who presented case studies of patients who improved their weight and health by eating in sync with circadian rhythms at the New York State Academy of Nutrition and Dietetics annual meeting in May 2016 explained:

> *"Because of circadian rhythms, there are variations in certain hormone levels, enzyme levels and glucose transporters at different parts of the day, which differentially affect how calories, carbohydrates and fat are metabolized. For example, research suggests that the calories we burn from digesting, absorbing, and metabolizing the nutrients in the food we eat, known as diet-induced thermogenesis, is influenced by our circadian system and is lower at 8 p.m. than 8 a.m."*[24]

Another reason why sleep affects weight is also related to the timing of eating. Research suggests that circadian rhythms could be a reason why many people who skip breakfast gain weight over time, even if they are eating comparable calories as those individuals who eat breakfast in the morning. An individual who skips breakfast and as a result eats their calories later in the day is out of sync with metabolic circadian rhythms and increases the risk for weight gain.[25]

If you work a night shift, you can re-sync your circadian metabolic rhythm by eating breakfast at the end of the workday, at 7 or 8 a.m., and then eat the heaviest meal when you wake up, about 3 or 4 p.m. The recommendations are to drink tea, eat vegetable soup, or if needed, snack on a small apple (in place of the optional after-dinner snack) to decrease overnight calories.

## Food Combinations

Another unique building block of my diet is the mix of protein, healthy fat, and fiber in meals and snacks. The mixture will help satiety (from protein and fat) and fullness (from high-fiber foods), clarifying that if you desire to eat outside the plan, it is due to reasons other than hunger such as boredom or stress. Although there are diets that dictate how to or not to combine foods, my way is proven through studies and clinically with my clients and myself.[26]

I refer to foods with "fiber," which is a nutrient, instead of indicating a food group, such as "carbohydrates," so that you have a wider range of choices for a snack. I admit it irks me when diets dictate to people that they *must* have three pieces of bread per day, for example. Let's say you don't want bread? As long as food has a natural source of fiber, such as a fruit or vegetable, it can technically count toward a snack portion.

The food combination also keeps your blood sugar stabilized. The glycemic index, or how quickly your body turns a food with carbohydrates into sugar, lowers when you combine carbohydrates with fiber, protein, and fat. The slow release of sugar decreases the risk of insulin resistance and causes you to feel fuller for longer, aiding weight loss efforts.

## The Differences in Snacks

In my 21-day plan, one snack will be a nut-based food with fruit, such as one tablespoon of almond butter with an apple. Another snack will be a non-nut protein such as one-quarter of an avocado, with non-starchy veggies including peppers, celery, and cucumbers. You can opt to add the non-starchy vegetables to any snack if you are still hungry because they are technically "free" on the plan; however, you cannot eat them within the mandatory 2-hour gap between eating. You can decide the timing of each snack, either in the morning or afternoon. There is also an optional after-dinner snack, which is one-half of a full daytime snack, such as one fruit. If you are under 5 ft. 3 in., over the age of 50, want to be stricter on the plan, or typically lose weight at a slow pace, it is advised not to eat after dinner.

Although cooking fresh is ideal, it is not always practical. I want your body and mind to become accustomed to less processed packaged foods that will eventually be a part of your life. There are "clean" bars that count toward a complete snack because they have the appropriate food combinations. Bonus: these snacks contain just enough sweetness to satisfy cravings and are convenient, allowing you to lose weight while keeping clean and kosher.

## Carbohydrate Rotation

My kosher girl's diet uniquely identifies the types and amounts of carbohydrates you can have per day. It is a common misconception that carbohydrates are only grains, such as bread. Because of the limited understanding of what foods make a carbohydrate, diets are either quick to forbid eating them because of their glycemic load or recommend overeating them due to their low caloric makeup. The problem is that while these diets may cause weight loss, the results are short-lived. At some point in life, if you are avoiding carbohydrates you will likely eat them. On the flip side, if you are on a diet that promotes eating mostly carbohydrates, you are probably overeating. According to studies, either scenario will leave you at the same disadvantage to sustainable weight loss by one year.[27]

My kosher girl's diet is different. Each day incorporates what I call a "carbohydrate rotation," to speed up weight loss and keep it off over time. For example, grains (e.g., oatmeal and sprouted whole grain bread), legumes (e.g., kidney beans and garbanzo beans) and starchy vegetables (e.g., sweet potatoes and beets) can be eaten as a portioned source of carbs once per day, separately in each of the three meals. The rotation of fiber-filled sources of carbohydrates maximizes benefits to your health, mood, energy, fullness, and weight loss on the plan.

## WHY CARBOHYDRATE ROTATION WORKS PHYSIOLOGICALLY

When I found the incredible effectiveness of rotating the source of carbohydrate in the day, I looked at science to figure out inherent properties within the category that make the strategy successful. Legumes (also known as "pulses") including lentils, chickpeas, and beans, aid weight loss because of their complex carbohydrates that include soluble and insoluble fiber. Pulses also contain resistant starch, which allows them to count toward a carbohydrate during a meal. Legumes also have satisfying protein, making them an option for protein as well, depending on how the meal is structured. For example, if you are eating grilled salmon as a protein in a meal and you also want legumes, they act as your carbohydrate and the serving size is ½ cup. Or you can choose to eat beans as a protein instead and then the portion size becomes 1 cup.

During the 1980s researchers discovered that you do not easily digest and convert all starches to glucose in the small intestine. Starches in legumes are resistant to digestion and pass to the large intestine where they are broken down by the healthy colon microflora. The subsequent research concluded that resistant starch functions in the body just as dietary fiber. Short-term experimental studies show that pulse consumption increases satiety over 2 to 4 hours, attributing these effects to the pulse carbohydrate composition. Additional studies demonstrated that regular consumption of pulses might be beneficial in weight management because of their nutritional composition: high fiber and protein contents, slowly digestible carbohydrates, and moderate calories.

Recently, a study was conducted to investigate the effects of bean consumption versus caloric restriction as a strategy to reduce the risk of metabolic syndrome: "The bean group was asked to eat five cups of lentils, chickpeas, split peas, or navy beans a week, and the caloric restriction group was asked to reduce energy intake." In other words, the bean group was asked to eat more food, and the calorie-reduction group was asked to eat less food. Not so surprisingly, the more-food group won. Not only was regular bean consumption as efficient as portion control in reducing pre-diabetes risk factors like slimming waistlines and better blood sugar control, but the bean diet led to additional benefits beyond calorie reduction, presumably due to some functional properties of the beans and peas. The researchers concluded that five cups a week of beans, chickpeas, split peas, and lentils in an ad libitum diet (meaning subjects weren't told to change their diet in any other way), reduced risk factors for metabolic syndrome. These effects were equivalent and in some instances stronger, than telling people to cut 500 calories from their daily diet. These results are encouraging news for individuals with or at risk for type 2 diabetes since they indicate that simple diet changes, such as the inclusion of beans, can have a positive impact on blood sugar control.[28]

Besides legumes, resistant starch is also present in the other three categories of carbohydrates on my plan including various grains and starchy vegetables, including plantains, potatoes, yams, corn, barley, and brown rice. It demonstrated that these foods have a beneficial effect in weight management by decreasing the blood insulin release after meals, thereby reducing fat storage in the cells. Also, consumption of foods high in resistant starch releases hormones that result in a decrease in appetite and increase in satiety, aiding in weight loss.

## Refocus Your Focus On the Scale

When I bump into people who have not seen me since I was pregnant or soon after I gave birth they frequently comment on how much weight I lost. While flattered, I quickly explain that although I lost my baby weight of about 44 pounds for the fifth time, I'm not at my lowest weight. I clarify that I'm at my fittest. With the Bioelectrical Impedance Analysis of InBody, I was able to track progress on the plan and uncover that I, along with my clients, lost fat, boosted lean muscle mass, and increased my resting metabolic rate. Results like these are what makes my weight loss more noticeable, more sustainable, and therefore, more worth it. It is easy to become addicted to a number on the scale and its natural daily fluctuations. However, similar to focusing on only the calories when reading a nutrition facts label, which only portrays a general picture, the scale does not tell the whole story about your weight loss success. There are many factors of weight including fat, lean muscle, skeletal muscle, water, and bone. My plan is guaranteed to cause fat loss, sustain or build lean muscle, and increase your metabolic rate, the actual factors that cause you to look slimmer and fitter.

Interestingly, for women over 50 or 55, it also results in water loss, which points toward the increase in water retention as you age. Men achieve faster results in fat and weight loss.[29] Women who typically lose weight at a slower rate may lose close to the 6-pound loss during the 21 days, yet they lose hard-earned pounds in the form of fat loss, not muscle, as is the case with most other diets.

There is no shame in giving yourself the necessary self-talk multiple times to drag your attention away from the scale. Consistently remind yourself that achieving a certain weight does not mean you will look the way you want. Weighing yourself is important in gauging a part of the success of the plan, but it is far from everything. Talking yourself through urges to constantly jump on the scale is what will help you resist and be more successful on your weight loss journey by boosting your morale and keeping your progress positive.

### Bottom Line on the Scale

During the 21 days, you will "check in" with your weight only one time per week during the phase of weight loss, and once per month during maintenance. I find that clients who weigh themselves more than once per week do not stick to one diet. An act that is seemingly innocent is another significant barrier to weight loss success. If the weigh-in is causing anxiety, throw the scale out altogether and gauge your progress by how you feel, measurements of your waist and hips, or pay attention to how your clothes fit. As I always say, no one imagines themselves feeling thinner than they are. We are our own worst critics. If you start to feel it, you are looking it. Appearing more fit and smaller in size is a better indicator of fat loss versus weight loss and muscle wasting, which leaves you looking drawn and bloated.

## Think "Limit," Not "Avoid"

Although this is a no-nonsense plan, it is not a no-food-group plan. My diet incorporates whole foods that are created by G-d and proven by science to be beneficial, but I am cautious about the processing and how much or how often I consume them. Food that may be tolerated by one person may not be best for another. Because of the rotation of foods on the plan, it is possible to identify sensitivities and intolerances. Food sensitivities can be a result of many things, such as having too much of one type of food. Once eliminated from the diet and subsequently reintroduced, a person can see if he or she experiences a reaction, or if eating something too often is the issue.

There is controversy in the industry between those who shame food groups like carbohydrates and fats, or nutrients like sugar, and others who will argue the opposite. My plan is "low" (not "no") in the controversial food groups of dairy, wheat (gluten), and soy because I rotate them within the week. You will not be eating every type of food group daily, but you will maintain balanced nutrition by consuming lots of vegetables, fruits, plant- and animal-based protein, and quality carbohydrate sources.

My plan is not technically an "elimination" diet, but a "rotation" diet. Because of the alternating food choices, some followers were able to identify food sensitivities. You should be aware of any feelings such as rash, hives, stomach upset, bloating, joint pain, fogginess, dizziness, and headaches while on the plan. Keep in mind, this diet isn't purposely meant to identify intolerances and you may or may not have a sensitivity regardless of the food plan.

Only note anything questionable or different that you feel in your Wellness Planner and see if a symptom pops up consistently, sometimes within three days after eating a particular food. Aside from the potential negatives, identify positive side effects experienced such as less bloating, better sleep, migraine improvement, more energy, and a general overall sense of feel-good vibes. If you are experiencing medical conditions such as skin issues, high cholesterol and high blood sugar, my kosher girl's diet will help as well.

## Treat Yourself

"The craving of him who lacks the opportunity to gratify it is much more intense than the craving of him who has such opportunity."

—TALMUD, YOMA 67A

As you read in the introduction, I lived and loved to eat, and I still do. You probably cannot name food I dislike, especially delectable treats including ice cream and chocolate. I never look to distinguish that flare of passion in my clients and I about eating, but to cultivate it in a way that truly allows us to enjoy the food by making it a mindful quality choice. I learned to anticipate a treat that is worth it, and ultimately the decision led to more enjoyment once I waited until a time I could focus and indulge.

I want you to love what you are eating. Think about it: after bite number three or after eating something for the sixth time that day, you truly stop tasting its deliciousness. After uncovering how much the "one treat a week rule" helped my clients and I not only lose weight but stay positive and enjoy the diet, it became a beloved part of my kosher girl's diet.

More than one Jewish client told me that the impactful strategy of knowing that the "treat card" can be whipped out during the week resembles a similar strategy in the Talmud called Pas Bisala. Pas Bisala is the story that involved a scapegoat being taken through the desert during Yom Kippur, a fast day, by the high priest. The lesson it teaches is a great tool that can help you commit to a diet. The priest had to walk a certain distance through the hot desert that day with the scapegoat to perform a commandment. The Talmud recorded that just in case the priest could not make it to the end of his journey because of dehydration or starvation it stated, *"AT EVERY BOOTH THEY WOULD SAY TO HIM, HERE IS FOOD AND WATER: Tanna taught: Never did anyone [who carried the goat away] find it necessary to use it, but [the reason of this provision is because] you cannot compare one who has bread in his basket with one who has no bread in his basket."* The section's opening quote originated from this Talmudic reference, *"The craving of him who lacks the opportunity to gratify it is much more intense than the craving of him who has such opportunity."*[30]

It may seem counterintuitive, but the Talmudic story teaches that if the food you crave is available and permissible, then you are less inclined to eat it. I have seen the same mindset work with my diet, even if we indulged on a portioned amount once per week. The strategy will help avoid veering off track by allowing yourself to feel less restricted while remaining in control.

Another significant aspect of the one treat per week rule is that if you slip and eat something "off" the diet, then you quickly catch yourself and write it off as your treat of the week. The rationalization instead of punishment is what will keep you motivated to move forward with the diet instead of spiraling down the slippery slope of binge eating on unhealthy options. My motto is that no one succeeds by being negative; a place of positivity achieves truly sustainable change.

Ideally, the indulgence is one serving of a clean treat from the recipes I provide in this book. You should consume the treat on a day and time that you feel the most in control of your food choices. For example, if nighttime is too much temptation, it may not be the best time to indulge. I typically say I don't get involved in people's choice of a treat or tell them when to eat it—that would defeat the whole point. Ultimately, the choice is up to *you* because *you* know *you* have control in something *you* feel you need to eat and enjoy, which causes *you* to be able to keep with the diet that makes the rule helpful. In other words: it is all about *you*. As a balance, swap out the protein in the vegetable snack when indulging on the treat and omit the optional after-dinner snack.

## GENERAL SUPPLEMENTATION

Bear in mind that one supplement does not fit all. The definition of a supplement means "in addition to" not "in place of" a quality whole foods diet. You should also be mindful that supplements have power, yet they are unregulated. Purchase trusted brands only (visit consumerlab.com) and never consume in excess or combinations that can potentially cause liver toxicity. Always talk to your primary care doctor before taking supplements, especially if you are on prescription medications and have a pre-existing medical condition. Here are my general supplement recommendations for most people:

1. Collagen powder
2. Vitamin D
3. Probiotic
4. Multivitamin
5. Quercetin or Turmeric
6. Other vitamins and minerals you identify as low or deficient through labs done by your doctor, such as B vitamins

## The Lowdown on Beverages and Hydration

I am known as the dietitian who loves coffee. Studies consistently show positive results to guiltlessly indulging in up to 3 to 6 cups of coffee per day. Keep in mind, this is talking about the standard 8-ounce size of pure coffee without added sweeteners, creamers, or syrups, or fancy names that sound like "frapa-wrappa-delta-camma-style" coffees. In fact, one reason I am a coffee fan, aside from the obvious benefits of decreasing stress, is because our palate is set up to enjoy the flavor of bitter.[31] If you enjoy bitter tastes, then it's easier to enjoy eating healthy foods. Think about the taste of most healthy foods such as vegetables: their flavor is bitter. Molding your palate onto the bitter end of the spectrum helps guarantee you won't be pulled back toward overeating processed, refined carbohydrates, aka "sweet foods" during the 21 days and beyond. Resetting your taste buds is another strategy that will finally help you break the cycle of yo-yo dieting because it will set you free of the sweet tooth anchor that keeps holding you down and away from long-term healthy eating.

## DAILY WATER NEEDS[32]

Method 1
- Weight: to convert your weight from pounds to kilograms, divide the number of pounds by 2.2
- 30-35 mL/kg of body weight for average adults
- Adult 55-75 years: 30 mL/kg body weight
- Adult >75 years: 25 mL/kg body weight

Method 2
- Dietary Reference Intakes: adequate intakes (AIs) for water
- Adult males (>19 years): 3.7 liters (L)/day (about 13 cups)
- Adult females (>19 years): 2.7 L/day (about 9 cups)

Because of the desire to like bitter foods, I am not a fan of using sweeteners, whether natural, manmade, alien-discovered, or something you concocted. My only pass is allowing one teaspoon or less of a natural sweetener, such as stevia or monk fruit extract, in something inherently bitter like coffee when you truly need it. However, you should try to skip it during the 21 days, and it may take you that long to acquire a taste for less sweetness. I also recommend you skip cow's milk in your coffee and grab the opportunity to incorporate a non-dairy alternative such as unsweetened almond milk, or my preference, unsweetened cashew milk, which has a creamier consistency in coffee.

If I had to pick one issue with coffee, it would be its addictive stimulant, caffeine. Although caffeine has its benefits, we coffee lovers are addicted. Addiction can lead to stress on the body and this kosher cleanse; we already established that stress and its parent hormone, cortisol, is something to avoid when the goal is to stimulate weight loss.[33] Personally, when I follow the 21-day plan for a reboot, I opt for a detox off coffee. I view the journey as an opportunity to break free of any chains tying me down to an unhealthy lifestyle in general. And, being honest, I sometimes feel the tension headaches, jitters, and insomnia, the negatives of caffeine sensitivity, if I go over my limit for the day. These symptoms are when coffee becomes a health no-no. People who either decided to keep their coffee a daily habit or kicked it out of their lives during the 21 days, resulted in weight loss on the plan. Honestly, I've had people on the plan who either kept their coffee habit, tweaked their coffee creation to include the non-dairy milk and no creamers, or skipped it altogether, and they all lost weight. However, the people who skipped the coffee completed the diet with greater mental benefits and an overall feeling of a physical and emotional reset and refresh.

## Ta, Ta, Tea

Before I leave you with the misconception that I completely skip my therapeutic moment of enjoying a hot beverage in the morning, think again. I begin each of the 21 days with a steaming hot cup of water with fresh lemon and mint leaves. The drink is what I call, "The Kosher Cleanse Elixir." You most likely heard of the recommendation to drink hot lemon water in the morning from the public. While there is no great science deeming it a miracle worker, I adopted it into my diet for my own reasons. During the night, after about 6 to 8 hours of sleep (or what you just learned your sleep will start to become if it is not there already), your body is dehydrated. The habit of waking up and drinking water is an excellent way to start your day and your metabolism. Adding the slice of lemon, while providing your body with more alkalizing benefits, also provides anticancer limonoids and antioxidants. Plus, adding the mint leaves (and tapping into my Moroccan roots), plants a layer of anti-carminative and anti-bloating properties targeting the stubborn belly bloat. It's that simple.

After drinking the Kosher Cleanse Elixir, I start on my Matcha Latte (see the recipe on page 97). Matcha is the whole leaf form of green tea in a powder. That means you get even more of the unique benefit of green tea, such as the anti-cancer property of EGCG and its correlative boosts for weight loss, with a "calmer" release of caffeine than coffee.[34] L-theanine is the most prevalent amino acid in matcha and is shown to have a relaxing effect on the mind and body with a boost in focus from the caffeine content. This effect may be because L-theanine increases serotonin, dopamine, GABA, and glycine levels in the brain.[35]

After the latte, I begin to drink my recommended 6-8 cups of plain water, sparkling water, flavored seltzer without artificial or natural sweeteners, or in the form of the Kosher Cleanse Elixir. While it is subjective how much water one needs in general (see sidebar Daily Water Needs on page 59), plus the addition of fluid content from the vegetables and fruit you consume, I recommend you focus on drinking water. Hydration is a key factor in your weight. Literally, it is one of the factors that make up your weight and a common reason why people plateau in or lack weight loss. Water was shown in two studies to boost your metabolism by also increasing your metabolism by 24 to 30 percent.[36] Don't let dehydration or inadequate fluid intake be the reason you are not successful at losing as much weight as you want. It is a silly consequence that is not even about the food we often focus on changing.

My obvious tip to ensure you keep drinking is to have a water bottle with you at all times. I enjoy using an infuser to add lemon and mint to the water. If you are having difficulty remembering, position the drinking time around your meals and snacks so that you reach your recommended fluid intake. Ideally, drink throughout the day, because your body needs fluids as you burn energy. It helps to mention that although it is annoying, a good sign of hydration is if urinating often, as long as the urine is a light yellow color, not dark or too clear. If you choose to drink a lot of water in one shot at night, for example, bear in mind that it may cause you to end up in the bathroom multiple times, and to lose weight you need your sleep too![37]

## Other Fluid Sources

Aside from matcha tea, other options such as anti-bloating green, mint, fennel, and chamomile, unsweetened, iced or hot, also count toward fluid and are encouraged to be sipped throughout the day, recommended at meal times, or used as something to hold you over at night. A 4-ounce serving of red wine is allowed in conjunction with what is or would be the Sabbath meals of Friday night and Saturday. If you drink wine, it counts as your optional after dinner fruit for that day. Otherwise, alcohol isn't advised during the 21 days but can be used the same way during maintenance.

**What to Track**

The morning of beginning the diet, take the following measurements and note them in your Metrics Tracker. Repeat the measurements at the end of the 21 days to report on progress. You will also need these parameters to decipher how many calories per day you need on the Daily Calorie Requirement calculations:

- **Weight:** Ideally use a medical scale. If it's electric, be sure you only go on one time and in the same location each time at the same time of day with the same clothes on. In other words, keep strictly consistent. You will only be weighing in one time per week, so that's three times total. Do not break this rule!
- **Height:** Note your height. You will need this number for your BMI calculation (see the BMI chart on page 64).
- **Waist:** Measure your waist right under your lowest rib and above your belly button. (Goal: <35 inches for females and <40 inches for males.)
- **Hip:** Measure your hip at the widest part of your buttock.
- **Waist to hip circumference equation:** Divide the waist measurement by the hip measurement to obtain the ratio. (Goal: <0.8 for females and <1.0 for males.)
- **Fat:** See Measuring Body Fat and BMI graphic below.

## MEASURING BODY FAT

### Body Fat for Men

- **Step 1:** Remove your clothing and use the bathroom when you get out of bed in the morning. Step on the scale to determine your body weight.
- **Step 2:** Use your last recorded height measurement at the doctor's office, or use a tape measure to determine your height in inches. Round up to the next inch if the measurement is over a half-inch. Round down to the previous inch if the measurement is less than a half-inch.
- **Step 3:** Measure your neck circumference. Look straight ahead. Wrap the tape measure around your neck underneath the Adam's apple. Keep the height of the tape measure level around your neck. Round up the neck measurement to the closest half-inch.

- **Step 4:** Measure your waist circumference. Stand tall. Place the tape measure around your stomach at the height of your navel and with contact against the skin. Breathe normally and record the measurement as you exhale. Round down the measurement to the nearest half-inch.
- **Step 5:** Repeat steps three and four three times for an accurate measurement. Add the three measurements together and divide by three to determine an average.
- **Step 6:** Insert your measurements into this formula: 86.010 minus (waist minus neck) / 100 minus 70.041 x (height / 100) + 36.76. The result determines your percentage of body fat.
- **Step 7:** Divide your bodyweight by the percentage of body fat to determine the number of pounds from fat weight.

## Body Fat for Women

- **Step 1:** Remove your clothing and use the bathroom when you get out of bed in the morning. Step on the scale to determine your body weight.
- **Step 2:** Use your last recorded height measurement at the doctor's office, or use a tape measure to determine your height in inches. Round up to the next inch if the measurement is over a half inch. Round down to the previous inch if the measurement is less than a half inch.
- **Step 3:** Measure your neck circumference. Look straight ahead. Wrap the tape measure around your neck underneath the larynx. Keep the height of tape measure equal around the neck. Round up the neck measurement to the closest half-inch.
- **Step 4:** Measure your waist circumference. Stand tall. Place the tape measure against your skin around your stomach at the thinnest part of your waist, usually between the navel and the breastbone. Breathe normally, and record the measurement as you exhale. Round down the measurement to the nearest half-inch.
- **Step 5:** Measure your hip circumference. Stand tall and place the tape measure around the widest part of your hips. Round down the measurement to the nearest half-inch.
- **Step 6:** Repeat steps three, four, and five three times. Add the three measurements and divide by three to obtain an average.

- **Step 7:** Insert the measurements into this formula: 163.205, (waist + hip, neck) / 100, 97.684 x (height / 100), 78.387. This is your body fat percentage.
- **Step 8:** Divide your body weight by the percentage of body fat to determine the number of pounds from fat weight.

Source: healthyliving.azcentral.com/calculate-body-fat-using-waist-measurement-weight-1389.html

| Description | Women | Men |
|---|---|---|
| Essential fat | 12–15% | 2–5% |
| Athletes | 16–20% | 6–13% |
| Fitness | 21–24% | 14–17% |
| Acceptable | 25–31% | 18–25% |
| Obese | 32%+ | 25%+ |

Table source: Health Check Systems, The American Council on Exercise

## Meal Exchange Lists

Although it is recommended to follow the meal plans and recipes correctly to ensure the proven results, it may simply not be an option for your lifestyle. You can follow along with the diet while making your meal options by sticking with the lists of foods in each category, their serving sizes, and the recommended frequency of eating them. You will also use this list to maintain your weight loss.

### Carbohydrates

*Grains*

*Nutrition:* 15g carbohydrates, 3g protein, 0 to 1g fat, 80 calories

- ▶ ½ cup, cooked whole grain: quinoa, high fiber cereal (+5g fiber), amaranth, whole spelt, buckwheat, Israeli couscous, brown rice, wild rice, black rice, red rice, pasta, farro, wheatberries, kasha
- ▶ Oatmeal, ½ cup raw, 1 cup cooked
- ▶ 1 to 2 slices Ezekiel bread or sprouted grain bread
- ▶ 4 whole grain Melba toast
- ▶ 3 thin rice cakes or 2 large rice cakes

## Body Mass Index Table

| Height (inches) / BMI | 19 | 20 | 21 | 22 | 23 | 24 | 25 | 26 | 27 | 28 | 29 | 30 | 31 | 32 | 33 | 34 | 35 | 36 | 37 | 38 | 39 | 40 | 41 | 42 | 43 | 44 | 45 | 46 | 47 | 48 | 49 | 50 | 51 | 52 | 53 | 54 |
|---|---|---|---|---|---|---|---|---|---|---|---|---|---|---|---|---|---|---|---|---|---|---|---|---|---|---|---|---|---|---|---|---|---|---|---|---|
| | Normal | | | | | | Overweight | | | | | Obese | | | | | | | | | | Extreme Obesity | | | | | | | | | | | | | | |
| | | | | | | | | | | | | Body Weight (pounds) | | | | | | | | | | | | | | | | | | | | | | | | |
| 58 | 91 | 96 | 100 | 105 | 110 | 115 | 119 | 124 | 129 | 134 | 138 | 143 | 148 | 153 | 158 | 162 | 167 | 172 | 177 | 181 | 186 | 191 | 196 | 201 | 205 | 210 | 215 | 220 | 224 | 229 | 234 | 239 | 244 | 248 | 253 | 258 |
| 59 | 94 | 99 | 104 | 109 | 114 | 119 | 124 | 128 | 133 | 138 | 143 | 148 | 153 | 158 | 163 | 168 | 173 | 178 | 183 | 188 | 193 | 198 | 203 | 208 | 212 | 217 | 222 | 227 | 232 | 237 | 242 | 247 | 252 | 257 | 262 | 267 |
| 60 | 97 | 102 | 107 | 112 | 118 | 123 | 128 | 133 | 138 | 143 | 148 | 153 | 158 | 163 | 168 | 174 | 179 | 184 | 189 | 194 | 199 | 204 | 209 | 215 | 220 | 225 | 230 | 235 | 240 | 245 | 250 | 255 | 261 | 266 | 271 | 276 |
| 61 | 100 | 106 | 111 | 116 | 122 | 127 | 132 | 137 | 143 | 148 | 153 | 158 | 164 | 169 | 174 | 180 | 185 | 190 | 195 | 201 | 206 | 211 | 217 | 222 | 227 | 232 | 238 | 243 | 248 | 254 | 259 | 264 | 269 | 275 | 280 | 285 |
| 62 | 104 | 109 | 115 | 120 | 126 | 131 | 136 | 142 | 147 | 153 | 158 | 164 | 169 | 175 | 180 | 186 | 191 | 196 | 202 | 207 | 213 | 218 | 224 | 229 | 235 | 240 | 246 | 251 | 256 | 262 | 267 | 273 | 278 | 284 | 289 | 295 |
| 63 | 107 | 113 | 118 | 124 | 130 | 135 | 141 | 146 | 152 | 158 | 163 | 169 | 175 | 180 | 186 | 191 | 197 | 203 | 208 | 214 | 220 | 225 | 231 | 237 | 242 | 248 | 254 | 259 | 265 | 270 | 278 | 282 | 287 | 293 | 299 | 304 |
| 64 | 110 | 116 | 122 | 128 | 134 | 140 | 145 | 151 | 157 | 163 | 169 | 174 | 180 | 186 | 192 | 197 | 204 | 209 | 215 | 221 | 227 | 232 | 238 | 244 | 250 | 256 | 262 | 267 | 273 | 279 | 285 | 291 | 296 | 302 | 308 | 314 |
| 65 | 114 | 120 | 126 | 132 | 138 | 144 | 150 | 156 | 162 | 168 | 174 | 180 | 186 | 192 | 198 | 204 | 210 | 216 | 222 | 228 | 234 | 240 | 246 | 252 | 258 | 264 | 270 | 276 | 282 | 288 | 294 | 300 | 306 | 312 | 318 | 324 |
| 66 | 118 | 124 | 130 | 136 | 142 | 148 | 155 | 161 | 167 | 173 | 179 | 186 | 192 | 198 | 204 | 210 | 216 | 223 | 229 | 235 | 241 | 247 | 253 | 260 | 266 | 272 | 278 | 284 | 291 | 297 | 303 | 309 | 315 | 322 | 328 | 334 |
| 67 | 121 | 127 | 134 | 140 | 146 | 153 | 159 | 166 | 172 | 178 | 185 | 191 | 198 | 204 | 211 | 217 | 223 | 230 | 236 | 242 | 249 | 255 | 261 | 268 | 274 | 280 | 287 | 293 | 299 | 306 | 312 | 319 | 325 | 331 | 338 | 344 |
| 68 | 125 | 131 | 138 | 144 | 151 | 158 | 164 | 171 | 177 | 184 | 190 | 197 | 203 | 210 | 216 | 223 | 230 | 236 | 243 | 249 | 256 | 262 | 269 | 276 | 282 | 289 | 295 | 302 | 308 | 315 | 322 | 328 | 335 | 341 | 348 | 354 |
| 69 | 128 | 135 | 142 | 149 | 155 | 162 | 169 | 176 | 182 | 189 | 196 | 203 | 209 | 216 | 223 | 230 | 236 | 243 | 250 | 257 | 263 | 270 | 277 | 284 | 291 | 297 | 304 | 311 | 318 | 324 | 331 | 338 | 345 | 351 | 358 | 365 |
| 70 | 132 | 139 | 146 | 153 | 160 | 167 | 174 | 181 | 188 | 195 | 202 | 209 | 216 | 222 | 229 | 236 | 243 | 250 | 257 | 264 | 271 | 278 | 285 | 292 | 299 | 306 | 313 | 320 | 327 | 334 | 341 | 348 | 355 | 362 | 369 | 376 |
| 71 | 136 | 143 | 150 | 157 | 165 | 172 | 179 | 186 | 193 | 200 | 208 | 215 | 222 | 229 | 236 | 243 | 250 | 257 | 265 | 272 | 279 | 286 | 293 | 301 | 308 | 315 | 322 | 329 | 338 | 343 | 351 | 358 | 365 | 372 | 379 | 386 |
| 72 | 140 | 147 | 154 | 162 | 169 | 177 | 184 | 191 | 199 | 206 | 213 | 221 | 228 | 235 | 242 | 250 | 258 | 265 | 272 | 279 | 287 | 294 | 302 | 309 | 316 | 324 | 331 | 338 | 346 | 353 | 361 | 368 | 375 | 383 | 390 | 397 |
| 73 | 144 | 151 | 159 | 166 | 174 | 182 | 189 | 197 | 204 | 212 | 219 | 227 | 235 | 242 | 250 | 257 | 265 | 272 | 280 | 288 | 295 | 302 | 310 | 318 | 325 | 333 | 340 | 348 | 355 | 363 | 371 | 378 | 386 | 393 | 401 | 408 |
| 74 | 148 | 155 | 163 | 171 | 179 | 186 | 194 | 202 | 210 | 218 | 225 | 233 | 241 | 249 | 256 | 264 | 272 | 280 | 287 | 295 | 303 | 311 | 319 | 326 | 334 | 342 | 350 | 358 | 365 | 373 | 381 | 389 | 396 | 404 | 412 | 420 |
| 75 | 152 | 160 | 168 | 176 | 184 | 192 | 200 | 208 | 216 | 224 | 232 | 240 | 248 | 256 | 264 | 272 | 279 | 287 | 295 | 303 | 311 | 319 | 327 | 335 | 343 | 351 | 359 | 367 | 375 | 383 | 391 | 399 | 407 | 415 | 423 | 431 |
| 76 | 156 | 164 | 172 | 180 | 189 | 197 | 205 | 213 | 221 | 230 | 238 | 246 | 254 | 263 | 271 | 279 | 287 | 295 | 304 | 312 | 320 | 328 | 336 | 344 | 353 | 361 | 369 | 377 | 385 | 394 | 402 | 410 | 418 | 426 | 435 | 443 |

Table source: nhlbi.nih.gov/health/educational/lose_wt/BMI/bmi_tbl.pdf

- ▸ 1 Wasa cracker
- ▸ 10 Mary's Gone Crackers
- ▸ 100% whole wheat, spelt, or kamut
- ▸ Whole grain rye crackers, 2 each
- ▸ Tortilla/pita-whole wheat, ½ large
- ▸ Tortillas-Low-carb, 2 small or 1 large
- ▸ Barbara's Original Puffins cereal 1 cup

## Starchy Vegetables

*Nutrition:* 15g carbohydrates, 3g protein, 0 to 1g fat, 80 calories

- ▸ Acorn squash, ½ cup cooked
- ▸ Beets, ½ cup cooked
- ▸ Butternut squash, ½ cup cooked
- ▸ Carrots, ½ cup cooked, 2 medium raw, 12 baby carrots
- ▸ Corn, 1 ear
- ▸ Parsnips, ½ cup cooked
- ▸ Potatoes, ½ medium Yukon Gold, new, or red potato
- ▸ Rutabaga, ½ cup cooked
- ▸ Sweet potato, ½ medium baked
- ▸ Turnips, ½ cup cooked
- ▸ Yams, ½ medium baked

## Legumes

*Nutrition:* 15g carbohydrates, 3g protein, 0 to 1g fat, 80 calories

- ▸ Beans, ½ cup: garbanzo, pinto, kidney, black, lima, navy, cannellini, mung, green soy beans
- ▸ Bean Soup, ¾ cup
- ▸ Hummus, ½ cup
- ▸ Lentils, ½ cup cooked
- ▸ Split peas, ½ cup cooked
- ▸ Sweet green peas, ½ cup cooked

*Non-Starchy Vegetables*

*Serving size:* ½ cup or 1 up for raw greens
*Nutrition:* Approx. 10 to 25 calories

- ▶ Artichokes
- ▶ Asparagus
- ▶ Bamboo shoots
- ▶ Bean sprouts
- ▶ Broccoli
- ▶ Brussels sprouts
- ▶ Cabbage
- ▶ Cauliflower
- ▶ Celery
- ▶ Cucumber
- ▶ Eggplant
- ▶ Garlic
- ▶ Green beans
- ▶ Greens: bok choy, escarole, Swiss chard, kale, collards, spinach, dandelion, mustard, beet greens
- ▶ Leeks, chives, onions, scallions, garlic
- ▶ Lettuce/mixed greens, romaine, red and green leaf, endive, spinach, arugula, radicchio, watercress, chicory
- ▶ Mushrooms
- ▶ Okra
- ▶ Radishes
- ▶ Salsa, no added sugar
- ▶ Sea vegetables (kelp etc.)
- ▶ Snow peas/Snap peas
- ▶ Squash, zucchini, yellow, summer, spaghetti
- ▶ Water chestnuts, 5 whole
- ▶ Shirataki noodles

### Oils and Fats

*Serving size:* 1 tsp., or as indicated
*Nutrition:* 1 serving = approximately 40 calories

- ▶ Avocado (fruit)
- ▶ Coconut milk (canned), light, 3 tbsp.
- ▶ Coconut milk (canned), regular, 1½ tbsp.
- ▶ Coconut oil (Organic)
- ▶ Flaxseed oil
- ▶ Ghee (clarified butter)
- ▶ Grapeseed oil
- ▶ High oleic safflower oil
- ▶ Mayonnaise (unsweetened, grapeseed or olive oil)
- ▶ Sesame oil
- ▶ Olive oil, extra-virgin preferable
- ▶ Olives, 8–10 medium

### Fruits

*Nutrition:* 15g carbohydrates, 0g protein, 0g fat, 60 calories

- ▶ Apricots, 4 whole, 8 dried halves
- ▶ Apples, unpeeled 1 small, 4 ounces
- ▶ Apples, dried no sugar added, 4 rings
- ▶ Applesauce, ½ cup unsweetened
- ▶ Banana, ½ large or 1 baby banana 4ounces
- ▶ Berries, blueberries, raspberries, blackberries-1 cup
- ▶ Cantaloupe, ½ medium
- ▶ Cherries, 15 cherries
- ▶ Dates, 3 dates
- ▶ Fried fruits, ex. Raisins, 2 tbsp.
- ▶ Fresh Figs, 2 figs, 3.5 ounces
- ▶ Grapes, 15 grapes
- ▶ Grapefruit, 1 whole grapefruit

- Honeydew, ½ of medium
- Kiwi, 2 medium
- Mandarin Oranges, no added sugar and juice removed, ¾ cup
- Mango, ½ of medium mango
- Orange, 1 large, nectarines-2 small
- Papaya, 1 cup cubed, 8 ounces
- Pear, 1 small pear
- Peaches/Plums, 2 small
- Persimmon, ½
- Pineapple, 1 cup
- Prunes, 3
- Strawberries, 1½ cups
- Watermelon, 2 cups

### Animal Protein, Grass-fed Ideally

Meat, poultry, and fish should be grilled, baked, or roasted; fish may also be poached. Keep cheese intake to 1 serving or less per day due to saturated fat, sodium, and intolerances.

- Beef, very lean (5% fat or less)
- Chicken, 4 ounces
- Cornish hen, 4 ounces
- Eggs, 2 whole or 3 egg whites plus 1 whole egg
- Fish, 4 ounces or ¾ cup canned in water
- Lamb, leg of lamb, 3 ounces
- Meat, red meat, 3 ounces beef-very lean (5% fat or less)
- Turkey, 4 ounces/6 ounces
- Cow's milk natural low-fat options: each serving = 15g carbohydrates, 8g protein, 0 to 3g fat, 100 calories
- Cottage cheese, nonfat or lowfat, ¾ cup
- Feta cheese, 2 ounces
- Milk, cows, 1 cup

- Mozzarella, part skim or nonfat, 2 ounces or ¼ cup shredded
- Parmesan Cheese (grated), 6 tbsp.
- Ricotta, part skim or nonfat, ½ cup
- Sour cream, nonfat, 6 tbsps.
- Yogurt, 6 ounces plain Greek/Skyr yogurt

### Plant Protein (Ideally Organic)

- Legumes (beans, chickpeas, lentils), 1 cup
- Avocado, 1
- Burgers, soy or veggie, 4 ounces
- Hummus, 4 tbsp.
- Nuts, raw, 1 ounce
- Tempeh, 3 ounces or ½ cup
- Tofu, 5-6 ounces or 1 cup fresh, 2-3 ounces cubed (baked)

### Dairy Alternatives

*Nutrition:* 1 serving = approximately 80 calories

- Almond milk, plain, 8 ounces
- Buttermilk, nonfat, 1% or 2%
- Hemp milk, plain, 6 ounces
- Soy milk, plain, 8 ounces
- Unsweetened coconut milk, 8 ounces in carton

### Nuts and Seeds

- Almonds, 15 whole nuts
- Chia seeds, 2 tsp.
- Coconut, unsweetened and grated, 3 tbsps.
- Flax seeds, ground, 1 tbsp.
- Hazelnuts, 15 whole nuts
- Pine nuts, 1½ tbsp.
- Pistachios, 2 tbsp.
- Pumpkin seeds, 2 tbsp.

- Sesame Seeds, 2 tbsp.
- Sunflower seeds, 2 tbsp.
- Walnut or pecan halves, 7 to 8
- Nut butter, 1 tbsp. made from nuts in this list

### Approved Extras: Condiments

- Coconut sugar, ½ tsp.
- Cinnamon
- Extracts, flavored, vanilla, almond, lemon, lime
- Green taco sauce, organic
- Herbs (fresh or dried), any, such as dill, basil, sage, thyme, rosemary, mint, chives, parsley, etc.
- Horseradish
- Monk in the raw
- Mustard
- Soy sauce (tamari)
- Spices, fresh or dried, any such as curry, paprika, chili powder, turmeric
- Stevia, 1 packet daily
- Tabasco sauce
- Tomato sauce/salsa, unsweetened
- Vinegars, unsweetened

### Beverages

*Intake:* 48 to 64 ounces daily

- Coffee (1 to 3 cups)
- Espresso 3 ounces
- Water (ideally filtered)
- Mineral water (still or carbonated)
- Tea, green, fennel, rooibos, unsweetened
- Herbal teas, non-caffeinated, mint, chamomile, hibiscus, fennel, etc.
- Seltzer, unsweetened

## Snack Exchange List

During maintenance, you have the flexibility to choose any option from the protein column and combine with any option under the fiber category to become one snack. Keep in mind what works for some people may not work best for you. If you feel you are not tolerating a food well or too much is increasing weight over time, choose another option or revert back to the snack options of the 21-day diet in order to get back on track.

### *Protein Snack*

- ▶ 1% Cottage cheese (½ cup)
- ▶ Light cheese stick (1 ounce)
- ▶ 0% Plain Greek yogurt (6 ounces)
- ▶ Hummus (2 tbsp.)
- ▶ Avocado (¼ fruit)
- ▶ Nuts, raw, unsalted (½ ounce): 10 cashews / 12 almonds / 14 peanuts / 8 walnuts
- ▶ Natural nut butter (1 tbsp.)
- ▶ Milk 0% to 1% fat (1 cup)
- ▶ Soybeans with pods (1½ cups)
- ▶ Low-fat Kefir (1 cup)
- ▶ Tuna (2 ounces)
- ▶ 1 hardboiled egg

### *Fiber Snack*

- ▶ Veggies (any non-starchy): cucumbers, celery, 8–12 baby carrots, etc.
- ▶ Fruit (any; for example): small whole fruit, berries (1 cup), melon (1 cup), mango (¼ cup), cherries/grapes (12), banana (½), grapefruit (½), ¼ cup dried fruit
- ▶ Light popcorn, 1–3 cups
- ▶ 100% whole wheat bread (1 slice)
- ▶ 6 Mary's Gone Crackers
- ▶ Rice cakes, 1 to 2 rounds

- ► Whole Wheat Wrap, ½ of a 9-inch wrap
- ► Whole Wheat Pita (¼ pita)
- ► Matt's Munchies, ½ package
- ► Kale Chips (2 cups)
- ► Tortilla Chips (10 chips)
- ► Granola, ½ cup

*Approved Snack Bars (the following count as a complete snack)*

- ► Kind Bar (<5 grams sugar, without soy protein isolate) ½ bar for 1–1,300 calories; 1 bar for 1,600+ calories per day
- ► Health Warrior Chia Bar
- ► Health Warrior Protein Bar: ½ bar for 1–1,300 calories; 1 bar for 1,600+ calories per day
- ► RX Bar: ½ bar for 1–1,300 calories; 1 bar for 1,600+ calories per day

  The following counts as ½ a snack and should be combined with another protein and counted as a "fruit:"
- ► ½ Larabar (or the 100-calorie snack size Larabars)

## Applicable Kosher Rules that Can Help Weight Loss

We already discussed the important specifics you need to know before shopping for kosher foods in chapter 3. Some kosher technicalities that dictate how and when you can eat are utilized in my kosher girl's diet as a method also to help you lose weight. Here are kosher laws that can be helpful for weight loss and the perceived difficulties will be easy to overcome:

### Kosher Guideline: You Cannot Mix Meat and Milk Together

According to kosher law and for this diet, you cannot combine dairy with meat foods. You should also store the dishes and utensils that are used to prepare milk and meat separately. You also cannot eat a dairy food within six hours after eating a meat one. Although it is not the reason for the law, by not eating milk and meat together you avoid eating calories from saturated fat, a known culprit that can cause weight gain and an increased risk of heart disease. The self-discipline of resisting putting dairy foods in your mouth after eating meat is an integral behavior to add to your repertoire of mindful-eating techniques that will help you lose weight.

### Kosher Guideline: You Cannot Eat Anything Not Inherently Kosher

Mindfulness and the strong will to turn down the food you simply cannot have is learned by keeping kosher. If food is not permitted to eat because it is not kosher, you provide the rationalization your mind needs to resist it.

### Kosher Guideline: Eat Meat and/or Fish at Sabbath Meals

Another helpful rule of my diet is that grass-fed red meat is offered once per week for Friday night dinner, relating to a kosher way of eating during the Sabbath. The allowance will help promote weight loss because excess red meat is associated with weight gain and poor health, yet in moderation, it allows for a mindful indulgence and a great source of iron and vitamin B12.

## What You Can Expect in the Next Section

Keeping kosher may seem complicated, but in actuality, it simplifies a weight loss diet. Now that you have the rules in place and understand the concepts behind my kosher girl's diet, you will start the actual 21-day plan in part 3.

### RACHEL'S STORY

*I decided to go on the Kosher Cleanse to jump-start a process of weight loss. I needed something very structured because, in the past, I always went off course in an attempt to lose weight. With each baby that I had, I gained more weight. Over the course of ten years, I kept gaining weight, and not losing at all! I guess I was too flexible with my food choices. The structure and rigid meal plan of the cleanse were exactly what I needed! I'm thrilled with the results! One thing I can say is that the recipes were delicious and I wasn't hungry, so there was no temptation to cheat.*

*My goal regarding loss was to lose at least two pounds a week while on the cleanse. After 21 days, I lost a total of eight pounds! My weight loss goal was successfully achieved and then some!*

*Here are some things that I learned from the cleanse:*

- *I can eat smartly and healthily, and feel satisfied and not hungry throughout the day.*
- *I can avoid sugar by substituting healthier sweeteners such as raw honey or a mashed ripe banana in almond butter muffins (delicious!).*

*What I enjoyed about the cleanse:*

- *The recipes are delicious and easy to follow! I feel like I bought a brand-new healthy cookbook!*
- *The menu was easy to follow, varied, and exciting.*

*What to keep in mind:*

- *Read the maintenance tips so that you can continue reaching your goal!*
- *Pay attention to the options of where to buy some of the harder to find foods. I was able to find a health food store near me that had most of the ingredients, so be sure to shop around!*

*Overall, I feel like I learned how to eat more smartly and healthily. I know that my food choices I'm making now are much better for my body and overall health, but I would still like to lose more weight and will continue another round of the cleanse!*

*Thank you for your guidance along the way. You and your team were very helpful and supportive!*

# Part Three
## GO!

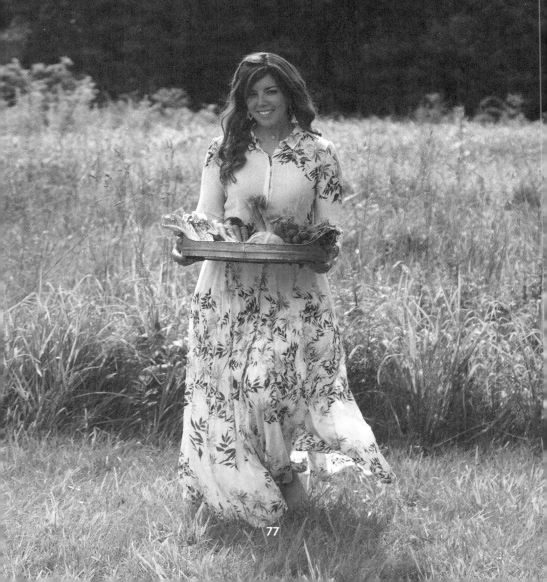

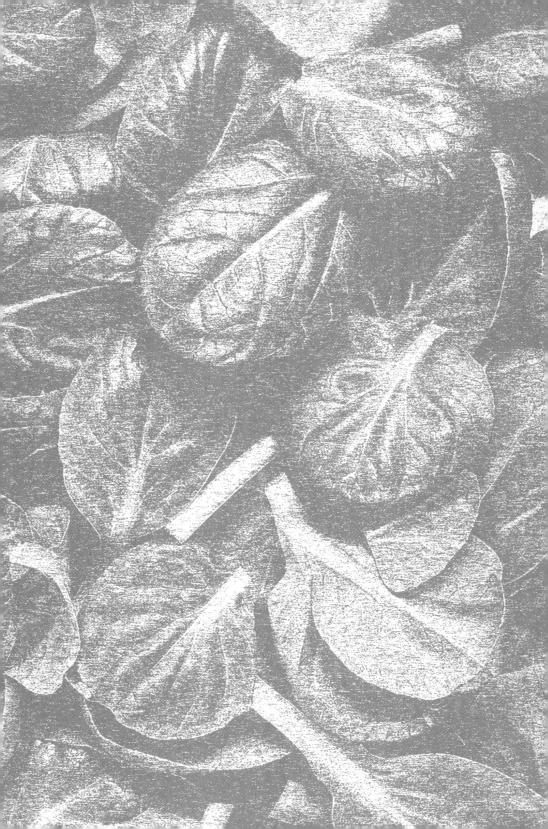

CHAPTER FIVE

# The "Diet" in Dieting with a Kosher Girl

## The Kosher Cleanse Protocol

You've prepped your mind, body, and pantry for clean, kosher cooking, geared yourself up with ammunition filled with rules and technicalities of my 21-day plan, and finally reached your last milestone: the actual kosher girl's diet. Each day you will recite an inspiring kosher quote to boost your motivation and serve as a spiritual self-affirmation. Then, after you drink the Kosher Cleanse Elixir, you will perform a recommended fitness activity. After that, you will move along to the scheduled breakdown of specific meals and snacks to create and eat, with accompanying recipes when needed.

## Nutrition Breakdown

The diet breaks down each day as follows:

- ▶ You will eat a portion of lean protein at each meal and a smaller portion of protein at each snack.
- ▶ You may eat an unlimited amount of non-starchy vegetables at all meals (see the Meal Exchange List on page 64), and you can add them to any snack.

▶ You may eat one serving of either a whole grain, legume, or starchy vegetable per meal as a carbohydrate, but only once per day of each type.

▶ You will be eating 2 to 3 fruit servings per day as part of a snack and/or breakfast.

▶ One snack will specifically be a nut-based food (e.g., almond butter) as the source of protein with fruit.

▶ The second snack will be non-starchy vegetable that's a source of protein that is not nut-based (e.g., avocado).

▶ There is an optional after-dinner fruit serving, if desired, but I do not recommend it for those with the goal of consuming under 1,800 calories per day (see the Daily Caloric Requirements on page 249 to calculate your needs), women over age 50, or those who have a history of unsuccessfully attempting to lose weight while following a plan, since this additional snack is a source of extra calories.

▶ You can add a non-starchy vegetable-based soup to each meal or snack if you are feeling too hungry (such as the Zucchini Soup recipe on Day 21).

▶ The menu includes the nutrients gluten, soy, and dairy 1 to 2 times per week or fewer.

▶ Kosher principles, such as not mixing dairy with meat, are at the forefront of the daily meal plans and only kosher foods are included. (I highlight further details in chapter 4).

▶ You may eat grass-fed red meat for Friday night dinner and Saturday lunch, only. Another lean protein may be substituted if you do not want to eat red meat.

▶ At least 8 cups of liquid per day are required, including unsweetened iced or hot teas (e.g., mint, green, and fennel).

▶ One serving of a mindful "clean" treat is recommended per week (see the recipes for Clean Treats on page 88) at a time of your choosing; however, the time to indulge should not be a typical time you feel out of control such as late at night. Choose to eat the clean treat instead of the nut-based snack that day.

## Other Daily Details

Each of the 21 days references a recommended exercise routine or is a dedicated rest day. You can follow the fitness images, links suggested at each day of the diet, or the Resources for Fitness on page 253 for realistic, moderate forms of physical activity to perform at any fitness level. The fitness recommendations incorporate a minimum number of steps per day and a kind of interval or resistance training. As discussed, over-exercising on the plan is discouraged as it will be counterproductive to the desired results.

It is important that you complete the Wellness Planner (see page 240) provided in this book each day. Your goal is to keep track of what you are eating and how you are feeling during the 21 days.

## Things You Need to Know Before You Start the BWN Kosher Cleanse

1. **The plan is low-carb, low-dairy, and low-gluten** with an emphasis on lean protein and fresh produce. You are decreasing your intake of highly processed foods. Every meal is homemade, but the preparation is simple if you follow the schedule recommendations, referred to as "Beth's Prep Tips." Aim to eat every 2 to 4 hours, beginning within 1 hour after you wake-up, up until 9 p.m. and at least 2 hours before bedtime. An example of a daily schedule is:

   - 7:00 a.m. Wake up
     –Mindful Meditation
     –Drink Kosher Cleanse Elixir
     –Fitness
   - 8:00 a.m. Breakfast
   - 10:30 a.m. Snack
   - 1:30 p.m. Lunch
   - 4:00 p.m. Snack
   - 7:00 p.m. Dinner
   - 9:00 p.m. Optional After-Dinner Snack
   - 11:00 p.m. Sleep

2. **It is important that you follow the meal plan** in order since most of the recipes are calorie and nutrient counted for a specific day.

If you want to swap a snack or meal from one day to another, it is advised to exchange an entire day within the same week. There is some prep to do the day before each challenge day, which will be indicated as "Beth's Prep Tips" so that you know how to prepare what is coming up.

3. **All of the weekday lunches and snacks are portable** so that you can take them wherever you need to go. You may have to create smoothies in advance to take out with you and keep refrigerated.

4. **I recommend going grocery shopping once per week.** Shop with the lists provided for each week on Friday, for example, and you will be prepared at the start of the next week on my diet. I recommend food prep for the week on Sunday and to launch the diet on a Monday, which is how I designed the 21 days in this book.

5. **Every serving of the fish, chicken, and turkey protein option in each meal is 4 ounces for women and 6 ounces for men**, which you may need to adjust when you see a recipe; otherwise, the serving sizes for the other food groups are the same for any gender. When eating red meat 1 to 2 times per week, the portion size for both men and women is 3 ounces. If you do not want to eat red meat, just substitute 4 ounces of either grilled fish or chicken. You can refer to the Meal Exchange List for recommended portion sizes of all foods.

6. **The ingredients in the recipes specify the amounts of salt.** Be sure to follow them to get the full results of weight loss. Other seasonings and ingredients that are unlimited are referenced in the section called "Free Ingredients."

7. **Keep in mind that you need to stay hydrated.** Your total fluid goals, including from foods, measure **about 9 cups per day for women and 13 cups per day for men**. There is no need to obsessively measure because fluid needs are subjective and you are consuming a lot of vegetables and fruit with a high liquid content, but most water glasses hold about 10 ounces. Therefore, about eight of those will get you to your goal.

The teas will help keep you hydrated, boost your antioxidant power to help detox, and aid de-bloating. They can be served iced or hot but always unsweetened. Feel free to include them with meals and snacks or anytime of day.

8.  **Ideally, no coffee or alcohol.** If you can't go 21 days without caffeine, try drinking 24 ounces (3 cups) of green or matcha tea per day or less. Be sure only to use one tea bag per cup or refer to the Matcha Latte recipe. Although I do not advise alcohol on the plan, red wine is offered as an option for Sabbath as designated on the menu and will substitute the optional after-dinner snack if consumed.

    You can opt to drink up to 2 cups of coffee per day, sweetened either with one teaspoon or less of stevia or monk fruit extract, with unsweetened almond milk or unsweetened cashew milk. Coffee does not substitute for any food or drink on the meal plan, and due to the goal of reprogramming the body not to rely on caffeine for energy, should be consumed when the stress hormone cortisol is at its lowest, between 10 a.m. to 2 p.m.

9.  **Ideally, you will be preparing some of the food you will eat for each week in advance.** But, life happens. If you find yourself having to eat out a couple of times, follow the guidelines at the end of the book on page 251, Eating Clean While Eating Out.

10. **Do not weigh yourself daily.** Weigh-ins are conducted once per week, at the same time of day and wearing the same clothes. Be sure to take measurements outlined in chapter 4 on the first and last day of the diet. Record the numbers on the Metrics Tracker included in this book.

11. **All meal plans account for macro- and micronutrient intake.** If you eat outside of this meal plan, you will not be following the diet to its fullest and cannot expect the same results. Stay true to your commitment and follow as precisely as you can.

12. **Exercise on the plan:**
    - 10,000 steps per day; track on your phone, with a pedometer, or a Fitbit.
    - Resistance/interval training: Look at the Resources for Fitness at the end of the book along with daily fitness links and guidelines to exercise 30 to 60 minutes on most days.

- You can exercise outside of these goals; however, bear in mind that your carbohydrate allotment does not account for rigorous aerobic activity. Be sure to schedule your training between a meal and snack time. For example, after eating a meal, exercise about 1 hour later, and after eating a snack, exercise about 30 minutes later. Position the next meal or snack to be eaten within 30 minutes after you completed your fitness for adequate recovery.
- I don't recommend performing physical activity at night during this plan because the nighttime eating recommendations do not account for optimal muscle recovery.

13. **Sweeteners:** Committing to a clean diet means eliminating added sweeteners, even the non-nutritive ones. Your goal is to reduce your sweet tooth by satisfying it with whole foods. If needed, you can add one tsp. of stevia or monk fruit extract to meals and snacks.

14. **Dairy:** Dairy is not tolerated by many people and is, therefore, rotated among other sources of protein during the week on the meal plan and not consumed daily. I do not recommend liquid cow's milk and soy milk on this diet as your first choice; instead, use the alternative milk listed on the meal plan (i.e., unsweetened almond milk, cashew milk, and coconut milk).

15. **Nutrition Breakdown:** My kosher girl's diet has an interesting use of carbohydrates. It defines a carbohydrate as any food with sugar and fiber (albeit different kinds of each). Because of that, the daily carbohydrate and nutrient breakdown for meals and snacks are as follows:
    - 1 whole grain per day
    - 1 legume per day
    - 1 starchy vegetable per day
    - 2 to 3 fruits per day
    - 1 nut-based snack with fruit/vegetable
    - 1 non-starchy vegetable-based snack with protein (other than nuts)
    - Optional after-dinner snacks of 100 calories or less of a whole food item such as one serving of fruit for those consuming a goal of over 1,800 calories per day

16. **EWG LIST:** I advise you eat as organic as possible on the diet. If you cannot commit to entirely organic ingredients, try to follow the EWG'S "Clean 15" and "Dirty Dozen" lists for those fruits and vegetables lowest and highest in pesticides. See ewg.org.

17. **Record a Daily Food Log/Mood/Fluid Diary** or Wellness Planner, even if you are following the meal plans exactly. Studies show you are more successful at consistent long-term weight loss if you keep a food journal[*] (read Lynn's story in chapter 6 to understand why).

18. You will often see indications to include "large salad" and/or "non-starchy veggies" throughout the 21 days. **The open options are meant to make the meal plan easier to follow by allowing you to choose how much you want to prepare.** It also allows you to include as many veggies as you need to feel full. Refer to the "Non-Starchy Vegetables" column on the Meal Exchange List (see page 67) as well as the images in this book for ideas on which vegetables to include during these times.

19. At times, you will see "grilled" or "roasted" without a recipe (e.g., "Grilled Chicken"). You can choose to season with approved seasonings (see "Free Ingredients") along with 1 tsp. of approved oil per serving, or copy the seasoning ideas from a different recipe.

## Beth's Prep Tips

 Throughout the 21-day program, I provide "Beth's Prep Tips" to help prepare you for upcoming days or provide a suggestion so that the diet is as easy to follow as possible. I recommend you start the diet plan on a Monday and make some recipes for each week on the preceding Sunday. Each day also includes suggested times of eating to keep the program easy to follow. Alongside individual recipes and days, I indicate if the yield will produce more than one portion to use at a later time during the 21 days or if you need to prepare a meal for the next day, such as Chia Yogurt, which has to be prepared the night before eating.

---

[*] Ingels JS., Misra R., Stewart J., Lucke-Wold B., Shawley-Brzoska S. The Effect of Adherence to Dietary Tracking on Weight Loss: Using HLM to Model Weight Loss Over Time. J Diabetes Res. 2017. Epub 2017 Aug 9.

Although it can be more work upfront, it is best to prepare and freeze the following items in advance. You can follow along with the "Beth's Prep Tips" within each day so that you are aware of what food and portion size are upcoming to defrost in time:

▶ Kale Pesto Sauce; freeze in an ice-cube tray as 12 (2-tbsp.) servings
▶ Gal's Black Bean Burgers
▶ Chicken Burgers
▶ Oat Apple Muffins
▶ Lentil Soup
▶ Butternut Squash Soup
▶ Zucchini (Vegetable) Soup
▶ Almond Date Balls
▶ Quinoa Crust
▶ Almond Butter Muffins
▶ Freeze cherries and grapes for optional after-dinner snacks

## Free Ingredients

Following is a list of ingredients that can be used at any time while on my diet to help season and flavor any dish, such as salads, proteins, and roasted vegetables:

▶ Balsamic vinegar
▶ Apple cider vinegar
▶ Mustard (be mindful how much you use due to its salt content)
▶ Sriracha sauce
▶ Spices—all (however, salt or blends with salt are not unlimited)
▶ Fresh lemon juice
▶ Naturally flavored and unsweetened seltzers, water, and teas
▶ Vegetable broth, no or low sodium
▶ No sugar-added sauces, ideally no or low sodium, from BPA-free cans

## Salad Dressing Recommendations

I recommend dressing pairings with each salad; however, you can use any of the dressing recipes below or oil-based dressings with approved clean ingredients. Feel free to adjust flavorings to your taste preference. I advise you to prepare a large amount of each dressing in advance and use about 2 tbsp. per serving throughout the 21 days.

### Honey Mustard Dressing

- ▶ 6 tbsp. Dijon mustard
- ▶ 6 tbsp. extra-virgin olive oil
- ▶ 2 tbsp. honey
- ▶ 3 tbsp. fresh lemon juice

### Lemon-Cumin Dressing

- ▶ 2 tbsp. extra-virgin olive oil
- ▶ Juice of 3 lemons
- ▶ 2 tbsp. cumin
- ▶ Salt, to taste

### Miso Dressing

- ▶ 6 tbsp. white miso
- ▶ 6 tbsp. sesame oil
- ▶ 12 tbsp. rice wine vinegar
- ▶ 3 tsp. grated fresh garlic

### Tahini Dressing

- ▶ 1½ cup pure tahini paste
- ▶ ¾ to 1½ cup of water to thin; more may be needed
- ▶ Juice of 6 lemons
- ▶ 1 tbsp. sea salt
- ▶ Chopped parsley, optional garnish

## Balsamic Dressing

- ▶ ¾ cup (12 tbsp.) balsamic vinegar
- ▶ 1 tbsp. garlic powder
- ▶ 1 tbsp. ground black pepper
- ▶ 2 tbsp. extra-virgin olive oil

## Clean Treat Recipes

The following are clean treats that approved at one serving per week. Clean treats should be a well-thought-out mindful indulgence to help keep your cravings at bay and maintain your positive outlook while following the diet. You may want to bake and freeze in advance, so you have them on hand when needed.

### CHUNKY BISCOTTI

Yield: 20 biscotti

**Ingredients**

2 eggs
1 tsp. vanilla
½ cup coconut sugar
1½ cups almond flour
¼ cup coconut flour
½ tsp. baking soda
¼ tsp. salt
½ cup unsweetened dried cranberries, optional
½ cup sliced almonds, optional
¼ cup semi-sweet chocolate chips, optional

**Directions**

1. Preheat the oven to 350°F.
2. In a large mixing bowl, beat together the eggs, vanilla, and coconut sugar.
3. In a separate bowl, mix the flours, baking soda, and salt until combined.
4. Combine the dry ingredients with the egg mixture while mixing slowly.
5. Fold in any of the optional ingredients you wish to include.
6. On a baking sheet lined with parchment paper, place the batter and form into a flat loaf.
7. Bake about 20 to 30 minutes until the top begins to brown. Remove and completely cool before slicing.

*Per serving (3 biscotti without optional ingredients): 140 calories, 9g fat, 1g saturated fat, 20 mg cholesterol, 180 mg sodium, 11g carbohydrates, 3g fiber, 5g protein*

## BLACK BEAN BROWNIES

Yield: 12 brownies

### Ingredients

2 (15-ounce) cans black beans, rinsed and dried well
4 tbsp. unsweetened cocoa powder
1 cup rolled oats
1 tsp. Kosher salt
¾ cup agave syrup
½ cup coconut oil, melted
4 tsp. vanilla extract
1 tsp. baking powder
⅛ cup chocolate chips, optional

### Directions

1. Preheat the oven to 350°F. Grease a 7x11-inch glass baking dish.
2. Combine all of the ingredients in a food processor.
3. Blend well for 5 minutes and until all ingredients are thoroughly combined, stopping periodically to push the batter from the sides. After its blended, use a spatula and fold in chocolate chips, if desired.
4. Pour the batter into the prepared pan. Bake for 18 to 20 minutes. Remove the pan from the oven and cool 8 to 10 minutes. Refrigerate so the brownies develop a firm texture.

*Per serving (1 brownie): 220 calories, 7g fat, 1.5g saturated fat, 80mg cholesterol, 130mg sodium, 0 carbohydrates, 0g fiber, 35g protein*

## ALMOND COOKIES

Yield: 12 cookies

### Ingredients

2 tbsp. coconut oil
3 tbsp. maple syrup
1 egg
1 tsp. vanilla extract
2 cups almond flour
½ tsp. baking soda
⅛ tsp. salt
½ cup chocolate chips, optional

### Directions

1. Preheat the oven to 350°F. Line a baking sheet with parchment paper.
2. Combine the coconut oil, maple syrup, egg, and vanilla and fold into the almond flour, baking soda, salt, and chocolate chips (if desired).

3. Scoop onto the baking sheet in the form of a ball and slightly press down into a cookie form.
4. Bake for 10 to 12 minutes.

*Per serving (1 cookie): 110 calories, 8g fat, 4g saturated fat, 15 mg cholesterol, 21 mg sodium, 6g carbohydrates, 2g fiber, 5g protein*

## CHUNKY COCONUT AND CHOCOLATE CHIP COOKIES

Yield: 8 cookies

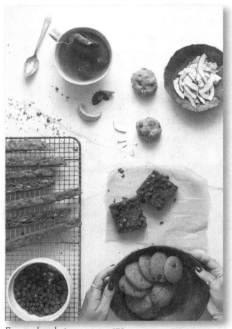

### Ingredients

2 tsp. vanilla extract
1 egg
4 tbsp. coconut sugar
½ cup coconut oil
1½ cups spelt flour
1 tsp. ground cinnamon
Dash sea salt
¼ cup coconut chips
¼ cup dark chocolate chips, optional

### Directions

1. Preheat the oven to 350°F.
2. In a medium mixing bowl, whisk together the vanilla, egg, coconut sugar, and coconut oil. In a separate bowl, combine the spelt flour, cinnamon, and sea salt. Whisking constantly, slowly add the dry ingredients to the wet ingredients.

*For a color photo, see page 170.*

3. Fold in the coconut chips and chocolate chips, if desired.
4. On a baking sheet lined with parchment paper, place scoops of about 1 tbsp. of the dough. Push down softly as the cookies do not rise high.
5. Bake about 8 to 10 minutes. Remove and completely cool before slicing. Place back in the oven for 5 minutes for a crunchier texture.

*Per serving (1 cookie): 150 calories, 11g fat, 9g sat fat, 15mg cholesterol, 5mg sodium, 11g carbohydrates, 2g fiber, 2g protein*

## OPTIONAL AFTER-DINNER SNACK

At the end of each day, you can choose to have an optional after-dinner snack. The snack is for those consuming 1,800 calories or more per day. If you are truly having difficulty curbing your cravings, it is better to mindfully consume one of these snack options at any daily caloric goal as opposed to ravaging through your entire kitchen cabinets and completely falling off the diet. However, please note that you will be adding calories to your day. The optional after-dinner snack should be less than 100 calories of one of our approved clean, kosher foods. If you are consuming them each night, rotate various options and avoid a "grain" carbohydrate. Aim to eat your after-dinner snack by 9 p.m. Here are some ideas:

- ½ cup unsweetened applesauce
- 1 small piece of fruit, or 1 cup of fruit, or ½ to 1 cup fresh fruit salad (depending on how small you chop the fruit and without added sugars or sweeteners; optional, add mint leaves for anti-bloating properties and natural flavor enhancement)
- 12 frozen grapes or cherries
- Non-starchy vegetables
- 2 tbsp. unshelled, unsalted seeds such as pumpkin or sunflower
- ½ ounce 70% dark (bittersweet) chocolate
- Baked apple: 1 small apple and1 tsp. cinnamon; bake at 425°F for 20 minutes.
- Smoothie: 1 cup of fruit and water, only

# Overall Recipes

Although I provide recommendations of which packaged products to buy that are clean and kosher in the shopping list, you may choose to create everything from scratch while you're on my diet. Here are some of my go-to recipes for many of the basics you will find throughout the 21 days.

## CASHEW MILK

Estimated yield: 1 quart or 4 cups

### Ingredients

¾ cup raw unsalted cashews
3 to 4 cups filtered water
1½ tsp. honey or agave nectar, optional
½ tsp. vanilla extract, optional
Salt to taste, optional

### Directions

1. Cover cashews with cold water in a large bowl. Soak for one hour or overnight.
2. Drain and rinse the soaked cashews.
3. Combine the soaked cashews and filtered water in a blender.
4. Blend on low, then slowly raise the speed to High for 1 to 2 minutes until the milk is completely smooth and no nut chunks remain. If desired, add sweetener, vanilla, and/or salt to taste.
5. Strain the milk through a fine mesh strainer, tea towel, or cheesecloth into a storage container.
6. Refrigerate the milk until it's thoroughly chilled. This usually lasts for 3 to 4 days if refrigerated.

(Recipe by Tori Avey)

## ALMOND MILK

Estimated yield: 2 cups

### Ingredients

1 cup raw almonds
2 cups filtered water

### Directions

1. Cover the almonds with about an inch of water in a large bowl. Soak them overnight or up to 2 days. (The longer the almonds soak, the creamier the almond milk will be.)
2. Drain and rinse the almonds.
3. Place the almonds in a blender and cover with the water.
4. Blend at the highest blender speed for 2 minutes.
5. Strain the almond mixture. Line a strainer either with the opened nut bag or cheesecloth, and place over a measuring cup. Pour the almond mixture into the strainer.
6. Press all the almond milk from the almond pulp (or "almond meal"). Squeeze and press with your clean hands to extract as much almond milk as possible. Store the almond milk in sealed containers in the refrigerator for up to two days.

(Recipe by Emma Christensen)

## WHOLE GRAIN SOURDOUGH BREAD

Yield: 1 loaf

### Ingredients

1 cup sourdough starter, fed and ready to use
1 cup plus 2 tbsp. lukewarm water
3 cups 100% whole wheat flour
2 tbsp. whole grain bread improver (for a better, faster rise), optional
1 tsp. salt
1 tsp. instant yeast
2 tbsp. vegetable oil

### Directions

1. Combine all of the ingredients, mixing until a shaggy dough forms (the consistency where you can pull a little off, but there is little to no gluten development so it is sticky and messy).
2. Let the dough rest, covered, for 20 minutes, then knead until it's fairly smooth and slightly sticky.
3. Place the dough in a lightly greased bowl, cover it, and let it rise until almost doubled in size, about 60 to 90 minutes.
4. Gently fold the dough over a few times on a lightly floured work surface.
5. Shape it into an 8-inch log, and place it in a 9 x 5-inch loaf pan.
6. Cover the loaf and let it rise until it's about 1 inch over the rim of the pan, about 60 to 90 minutes. Towards the end of the rising time, preheat the oven to 350°F.
7. Bake 40 to 45 minutes, or until the loaf is golden brown and a digital thermometer inserted into the center registers 205°F to 210°F. Remove the bread from the oven, let it sit in the pan for 5 minutes, then turn it out onto a rack to cool.

(Recipe by kingarthurflour.com)

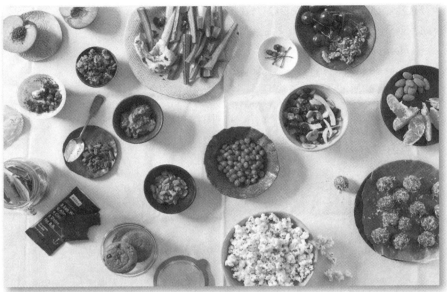

*For a color photo, see page 172-173.*

## GREEK YOGURT

### *Ingredients*

1 liter (¼ gallon) of milk
3 tbsp. live yogurt or one yogurt starter package
Cheesecloth

### *Directions*

1. Pour the milk into a saucepan and heat over medium-high until it is nearly scalding. When it reaches a temperature of about 176°F, remove it from the heat.
2. Let the milk cool to a temperature of 108° to 115°F. Transfer it to a glass bowl, and allow to cool until it's just warm to the touch.
3. After the milk has cooled until it's just warm, whisk in the live yogurt or one yogurt starter package until it's completely incorporated.
4. Cover the mixture with a clean towel, turn the oven to its warm setting, and let rest at least 4 hours but preferably overnight. If possible, set the oven temperature so that it stays at a steady 108°F for the entire time.
5. Strain the yogurt. After a while, the yogurt should look like a white firm custard. Place the cheesecloth muslin cloth into a sieve with a glass bowl placed underneath. Ladle the yogurt into the cloth and allow it to strain, until it achieves your desired consistency. When your yogurt has reached the consistency that you wish, it is ready to serve.

(Recipe by makegreekyogurt.com)

## GUACAMOLE

### Ingredients

2 ripe avocados
½ tsp. Kosher salt
1 tbsp. fresh lime or lemon juice
2 tbsp. chopped red onion
2 tbsp. finely chopped cilantro
Dash freshly ground black pepper
1 to 2 serrano chilies, stems and seeds removed, minced
1 tomato, seeds and pulp removed, chopped

### Directions

1. Cut the avocados in half and remove the pit. Score the inside of the avocado, scoop out the flesh with a spoon, and place in a bowl.
2. Using a fork, roughly mash the avocados, but do not overdo it.
3. Sprinkle the avocados with salt and lime or lemon juice. Add the onion, cilantro, black pepper, and chilies. Adjust the amount of chili peppers to your preferred spiciness.
4. Cover with plastic wrap and chill to store. (Chilling tomatoes hurts the guacamole flavor, so if you desire chopped tomatoes, add it before serving.)

(Recipe by Elise Bauer)

## HUMMUS

Yield: 6 servings or about 1½ cups

### Ingredients

¼ cup fresh lemon juice or the juice of 1 large lemon
¼ cup well-stirred tahini
1 to 2 small garlic cloves, minced
2 tbsp. extra-virgin olive oil, plus additional for serving
½ tsp. ground cumin
Salt to taste
1½ cups cooked chickpeas, drained and rinsed
2 to 3 tbsp. water
Dash ground paprika, for serving

### Directions

1. Into a food processor, combine the lemon juice and tahini and process for 1 minute. Scrape the sides and bottom of the bowl; process for 30 seconds more.
2. Add the olive oil, garlic, cumin, and ½ tsp. salt to the tahini-lemon juice mixture. Process for 30 seconds, scraping the sides and bottom of the bowl; process another 30 seconds.

(recipe continues, page 96)

3. Add half of the chickpeas to the food processor and process for 1 minute. Scrape the sides and bottom of the bowl, add remaining chickpeas, and process until thick and quite smooth, about 1 to 2 minutes.
4. If the hummus too thick or still has tiny bits of chickpeas, with the food processor on, slowly add water until you reach the perfect consistency.
5. Taste for salt and adjust as needed. Serve with a drizzle of olive oil and dash of paprika.

(Recipe by inspiredtaste.net)

# Flours
## ALMOND FLOUR
You will need a food processor or high RPM blender for this recipe.

### Ingredients
1 cup almonds

### Directions
1. Place the almonds into a food processor or blender.
2. Secure the lid and place the tamper inside the blender, if using a blender. (Use the tamper if necessary to get almonds moving.)
3. Turn blender on high (for a Vitamix use High, Speed 10) for 7 seconds. Done!

(Recipe by: Hollie Jeakins)

## OAT FLOUR
You will need a food processor or high RPM blender for this recipe.

### Ingredients
1 cup rolled or old-fashioned oats

### Directions
1. Place the oats into the bowl of a food processor or blender.
2. Pulse the oats until ground into a powder-like consistency. Depending on the speed and power of your food processor or blender, this should take 60 seconds or less.
3. Stop the machine and stir to ensure that all the oats finely ground. Store unused portions in an airtight container.
4. One cup of rolled oats yields approximately 1 cup of oat flour.

(Recipe by Alison Bickel, "Momables." Bickel, A. How to Make Oat Flour. Retrieved September 25, 2017 from momables.com/how-to-make-oat-flour/)

## QUINOA FLOUR

You will need a clean coffee bean grinder for this recipe.

### Ingredients

2 cups organic quinoa

### Directions

1. Rinse quinoa through a fine-mesh sieve for about 1 minute and then dry quinoa.
2. Preheat the oven to 350°F.
3. On an ungreased rimmed baking sheet, bake the quinoa for 12 to 15 minutes until dry, slightly golden, and fragrant; cool completely.
4. Put about ¼ cup of the quinoa seeds into the coffee grinder, and pulse to grind. Shake the grinder every few pulses to ensure an even grind. Repeat until all of the quinoa is finely ground.

(Author: Peace. Love. Quinoa. peacelovequinoa.com/2015/1½7/quinoa-flour-diy/)

# Drinks

## KOSHER CLEANSE ELIXIR

### Ingredients

1 cup water (hot or cold)
½ lemon
Fresh mint

### Directions

Squeeze the lemon juice into the water and then add mint leaves.

## MATCHA LATTE

### Ingredients

¾ cup unsweetened almond milk or unsweetened cashew milk
1 tsp. Matcha powder
Boiling water
1 tsp or packet of stevia or monk fruit extract, optional

### Directions

1. In a small pot, heat the almond or cashew milk over medium-high heat until it's just simmering.
2. Place the matcha powder in a heatproof cup. Slowly whisk in ¼ cup boiling water and then the milk, tipping the cup slightly to create foam. Add sweetener, if desired. (You can also use a frother to foam your milk.)

*Per serving: 37 calories, 3g carbohydrates, 2g fat, 1g protein, 136mg sodium*

(Recipe by Christine Muhlke. Muhlke, C. Matcha Latte. February 2013. Retrieved on September 25, 2017 from bonappetit.com/recipe/matcha-latte)

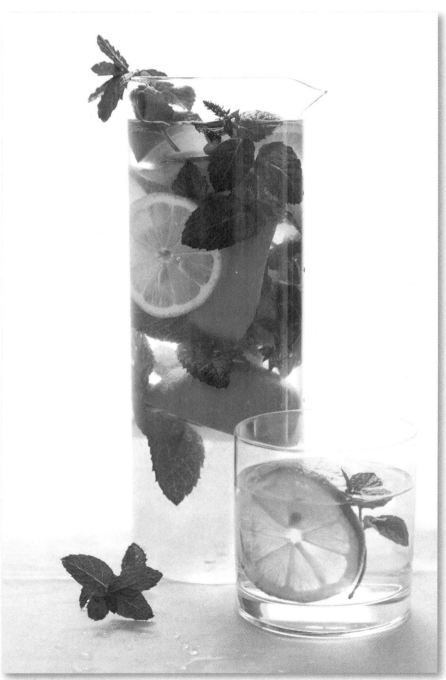

For a color photo, see page 171.

# The Start

*"A man is led the way he wishes to follow."*

—TALMUD, MAKKOTH 10B

You've made it to the diet! Always remember that your commitment to achieve personal health and weight goals led you to my 21-day kosher girl's diet. I will guide you each day with an inspiring quote like this one from the Talmud to remind you of why you are here, keep you focused and help set your daily intention. I hope that my favorite "kosher motivations" give you the boost you need in times of struggle and on the contrary, amplifies positive vibes when you are feeling motivated. Get ready for an exhilarating journey for your mind and body.

It's weigh-in day! Plus, it is time to take all the other metrics to measure including, waist, hip, and body fat. Note them all in your Weight Tracker.

## BETH'S PREP TIP

Don't forget it's Sunday! Make sure to prepare your snacks and the recommended parts of your meal to make in advance!

# DAY ONE

## Mindful Meditation to Start Your Day

*"If I am not for me, who is for me; and if I am (only) for myself, what am I. And if not now, when?"*

—HILLEL, ETHICS OF THE FATHERS 1:14

*"I find this to be the most inspirational and motivating message. I was created for a specific purpose—there is no other 'me.' Consider that I am here for others—bearing the 'me' in mind, how can I make the difference to the world? Lastly, there's no time like the present."*

—RABBI CHAIM COHEN

WELCOME! You shopped and prepped your clean kosher foods. You studied and learned all there is to know about keeping a clean and kosher diet. You committed your mind and body to transform into your best self. You are motivated to pursue your passion and enhance your health while reaching ideal weight loss. Today's quotes teach that there is no time like the present and there is no one who can get you to your goal but you. You have the power. Turn the page and get started!

## For Starters

 **Kosher Cleanse Elixir:** Drink upon waking (see page 97).

 **Daily Fitness Goal:** Ease into the diet for 15 minutes with a boost of motivation and physical fitness from your choice of yoga routine, such as shown in this "Power Yoga" video (youtube.com/watch?v=tFk7SVtjs38). Don't forget to walk your 10,000 steps today!

## Breakfast

• **Berry Oatmeal**

## Snack

• ½ medium grapefruit with 10 raw cashews

## Lunch

• 1 cup unsweetened green tea, hot or iced
• 1 large salad that includes any non-starchy veggies and ½ cup kidney beans with 4 ounces grilled wild salmon (or 1 can wild salmon)
• Suggested dressing: 2 tbsp. **Lemon-Cumin Dressing**

## Snack

• 2 or more Persian cucumbers with **Avocado Mash**

## Dinner

• 1 cup unsweetened fennel tea, hot or iced
• 2 **Chicken Burgers** with **Brussel Sprouts** and ½ cup **Beet Salad**

### BETH'S PREP TIPS

• I like to add the berries to the oatmeal as it is cooking, but you can add the fruit after the oatmeal is cooked.
• Freeze the extra salmon. On Days 3, 9, 11, and 21 you will be having 4 ounces of salmon in various ways.
• Freeze the extra **Chicken Burgers** for Day 17.
• Freeze the leftover **Brussels Sprouts**. You will have them again on Day 15.

# Day One Recipes

## BERRY OATMEAL

Yield: 1 serving

### Ingredients

½ cup rolled oats
¼ cup unsweetened almond milk
½ cup "tri-berries" (blueberries, raspberries, and blackberries)
1 tsp. chia seeds
1 tsp. vanilla extract

### Directions

1. Cook oatmeal in the almond milk as directed by the package.
2. Add the chia seeds, vanilla, and tri-berries to a bowl.

*Per serving: 220 calories, 5g fat, 0.5g saturated fat, 0mg cholesterol, 45mg sodium, 38g carbo-hydrates, 8g fiber, 6g protein*

## AVOCADO MASH

### Ingredients

¼ avocado
Lemon juice, to taste
Red pepper flakes and ground cumin, optional

### Directions

1. Mash the avocado.
2. Add seasonings such as the red pepper flakes and cumin, if desired, with a splash of lemon for a boost of flavor.

*Per serving: 80 calories, 7g fat, 1g saturated fat, 0mg cholesterol, 0g sodium, 4g carbohydrates, 3g fiber, 1g protein*

## CHICKEN BURGERS

Yield: 6 chicken burgers

### Ingredients

1 lb. ground white meat chicken
2 tbsp. extra-virgin olive oil
1 small onion, finely chopped
½ yellow or orange bell pepper, seeded and chopped
1 handful spinach leaves, finely chopped, or ¼ cup frozen chopped spinach, defrosted
1 celery stalk, finely chopped
Coarse salt and ground pepper, to taste
1 tbsp. Dijon mustard

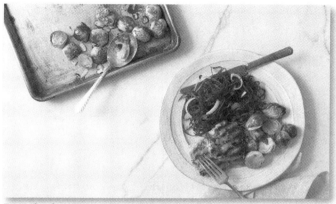

*For a color photo, see page 174-175.*

### Directions

1. Combine all ingredients in a bowl.
2. Form into burger shapes to make 6 patties.
3. Grill on a grill pan about 4 minutes per side, or bake in the oven on a baking sheet for about 12 minutes on 350°F.

*Per serving (1 burger): 170 calories, 11g fat, 2.5g saturated fat, 65mg cholesterol, 180mg sodium, 3g carbohydrates, 0.83g fiber, 14g protein*

## BRUSSELS SPROUTS

Yield: 4 servings

### Ingredients

2 cups Brussels sprouts, sliced in half (if frozen, defrost first)
1 tbsp. extra-virgin olive oil
¼ cup sliced almonds, toasted
Juice of 1 lemon
1 tsp. onion powder
Salt and pepper, to taste

### Directions

1. Preheat the oven to 425°F.
2. Line a baking sheet with parchment paper. Place the Brussels sprouts in one layer onto the sheet. Drizzle the olive oil over the Brussels sprouts and toss to coat.
3. Roast about 30 minutes (you may want to toss the sprouts, or flip them after about 15 minutes for even roasting).
4. Add the almonds, lemon, onion powder, and salt and pepper, and stir to combine.

*Per serving (about ½ cup): 90 calories, 7g fat, 0.5 saturated fat, 0mg cholesterol, 10mg sodium, 6g carbohydrates, 3g fiber, 3 g protein*

## BEET SALAD

Yield: 2 servings

### Ingredients

4 beets
½ tsp. ground cumin
½ tsp. salt
½ tsp. pepper
1 tsp. apple cider vinegar
1 red onion, chopped

### Directions

1.  Place the beets in a high-sided dish in the oven on 350°F, covered halfway with water, and cook about an hour and a half until they're soft. Remove from the oven and cool.
2.  Rub off the skin of the beets (use gloves!) and cut into cubes.
3.  Season with the cumin, salt, pepper, and apple cider vinegar.
4.  Add the onion to the beet mixture.
5.  Stir to combine.

*Per serving: 90 calories, 0g fat, 0g saturated fat, 0mg cholesterol, 575mg sodium, 21g carbohydrates, 5g fiber, 3g protein*

# DAY TWO

## Mindful Meditation to Start Your Day

*"Rabbi Tarfon says: you are not obligated to finish the work;*
*nor are you free to desist from it."*

—ETHICS OF THE FATHERS 2:21

Rabbi Tarfon was referring to the study of the *Torah* (Old Testament) and the obligation to continue throughout one's life to "repair/perfect the world" (referred to in Hebrew as *Tikkun Olam*). I interpret it as a good rule of thumb for life in general, too. Simply put: never give up no matter how tough the journey. No one is forcing you to finish; however, you have an obligation to yourself to see through your commitment. Remember, you chose to diet because you believed in yourself and felt a desire to change your status quo. Do not quit because you are giving up on yourself. You have the strength to make it to the end of the 21 days. Quickly jot down three motivators of why you decided to follow my diet, read them out loud, hang them up on your refrigerator to refer back to daily and then keep on going!

## For Starters

 **Kosher Cleanse Elixir:** Drink upon waking (see page 97).

 **Daily Fitness Goal:** Aside from walking your 10,000 steps today, pump up the volume of your workout with this HIIT Total Body Workout for Beginners (youtube.com/watch?v=-_tJ1Se57WE).

## Breakfast

- **Anti-Inflammatory Omelet** with diced non-starchy veggies and 1 pear

## Snack

- 1 small orange with 12 raw almonds

## Lunch

- 1 cup unsweetened fennel tea, hot or iced
- 1 cup **Quinoa Salad** with 2 tbsp. **Lemon-Cumin Dressing**

## Snack

- 2 tbsp. **Hummus** with 1 medium carrot

## Dinner

- 1 cup unsweetened fennel tea, hot or iced
- 4 ounces **Zaatar Branzini** with 1 **Roasted Eggplant Tahini Drizzle** and **Roasted Sweet Potatoes**

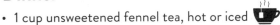 **BETH'S PREP TIPS**

- Keep the leftover hummus in an airtight container to be used later on during the 21 days. If it is not an option to make your own hummus, you can purchase store-bought brands of classic hummus, or the snack-sized varieties.
- Be sure to freeze the extra 4 ounces of branzini for Day 21. You can substitute another whitefish, except tilapia, for the branzini.

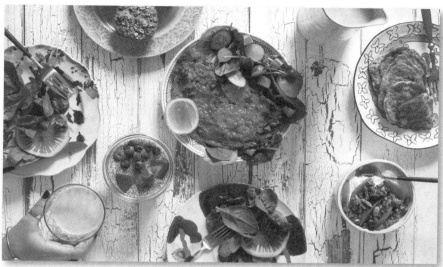

*For a color photo, see page 178.*

# Day Two Recipes

## ANTI-INFLAMMATORY OMELET

Yield: 1 serving

### Ingredients

2 egg whites plus 1 whole egg
Salt and black pepper, to taste
1 tbsp. extra-virgin olive oil
⅛ tsp. turmeric
2 scallions, finely chopped, white and light green parts only
¼ cup diced tomato

### Directions

1. Whisk together the eggs, salt, and pepper. Set aside.
2. Heat the olive oil in a large skillet (ideally cast-iron) over medium-high heat. Add the scallions and turmeric.
3. Cook 30 seconds or until the scallions soften, stirring often.
4. Add the tomato and cook about 1 minute, stirring frequently.
5. Pour the egg mixture into the pan. Swirl the mixture so that it spreads evenly.
6. Cook about 2 minutes until the edges of the egg mixture start to brown; flip to cook the other side.

*Per serving: 250 calories, 18g fat, 3.5g saturated fat, 195mg cholesterol, 290mg sodium, 6g carbohydrates, 2g fiber, 13g protein*

## QUINOA SALAD

Yield: 4 servings

### Ingredients

½ cup uncooked quinoa, cooked according to package directions
½ cup black beans, rinsed
1 red, orange, and yellow bell pepper, seeded and chopped
½ cup organic corn niblets
2 tbsp. chopped fresh parsley

### Directions

1. In a large bowl, combine the quinoa, black beans, bell peppers, corn, and parsley.
2. Pair with 2 tbsp. **Lemon-Cumin Dressing** per serving.

*Per serving: 140 calories, 1.5g fat, 95g carbohydrates, 0g saturated fat, 0mg cholesterol, 200mg sodium, 5g fiber, 6g protein*

## ZAATAR BRANZINI

Yield: 1 serving

### Ingredients

4 ounces branzini fillet (or any lean whitefish fillet, except tilapia)
1 tbsp. extra-virgin olive oil
1 tsp. zaatar spice
Juice of ½ lemon

### Directions

1. Marinate the fish in the seasonings (oil, zaatar, and lemon juice). Refrigerate 1 hour, ideally.
2. Preheat the oven to 350°F.
3. Line a baking sheet with parchment paper. Place each fish fillet on the baking sheet.
4. Bake for 12 minutes.

*Per serving: 230 calories, 16g fat, 2g saturated fat, 0mg cholesterol, 75mg sodium, 2g carbohydrates, 0g fiber, 21g protein*

## ROASTED SWEET POTATOES

Yield: 1 serving

### Ingredients

½ cup cubed sweet potatoes
1 tsp. extra-virgin olive oil
Paprika
Garlic powder
Salt and pepper, to taste

### Directions

1. Preheat the oven to 425°F.
2. Place sweet potatoes in a bowl and toss in the olive oil and seasonings (paprika, garlic powder, salt, and pepper) to coat.
3. Spread the potatoes in one layer on a baking sheet lined with parchment paper.
4. Roast about 30 minutes or until desired crispness, turning the sweet potatoes in the middle of roasting for even cooking.

*Per serving: 111 calories, 5g fat, 0.5g saturated fat, 0mg cholesterol, 155mg sodium, 16g carbohydrates, 2g fiber, 1g protein*

## ROASTED EGGPLANT TAHINI DRIZZLE

Yield: 4 servings

### Ingredients

2 eggplants, halved and scored
    in a crisscross pattern
¾ tsp. Kosher salt
½ tsp. black pepper
1 tsp. garlic powder
2 tsp. extra virgin olive oil
2 tbsp. **Tahini Dressing**
½ cup pomegranate seeds
4 tbsp. white chia seeds
Parsley, for garnish, optional

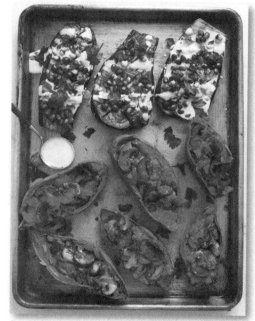

### Directions

1. Preheat the oven to 350°F.
2. Rub the salt, pepper, garlic powder, and extra-virgin olive oil on the eggplants.
3. Bake for 35 to 50 minutes depending on eggplant thickness until soft and tender.

*For a color photo, see page 179.*

4. Drizzle the tahini on all halves (see **Tahini Dressing**).
5. Sprinkle the pomegranate and white chia seeds on all halves. Garnish with parsley, if desired.

*Per serving: 180 calories, 8g fat, 1g saturated fat, 0mg cholesterol, 237mg sodium, 25g carbohydrates, 12g fiber, 6g protein*

# DAY THREE

## Mindful Meditation to Start Your Day

*"Shimon (son of Rabban Gamliel) says:*
*It is not what one says, but rather what one does,*
*that makes all the difference in the world."*
—ETHICS OF THE FATHERS 1:17

Most people can talk the talk, but you are walking the walk! Check out the way you fiercely woke up this morning, ready to put yourself first with your actions, not only your words. Bask in the incredible glory from taking more steps towards your ideal weight. There are not many motivators as good as feeling empowered both physically and emotionally. By starting your day and following the fitness routine along with the beverage, snacks, and meal options you are taking the actions needed to make a difference in your world!

## For Starters

 **Kosher Cleanse Elixir:** Drink upon waking (see page 97).

 **Daily Fitness Goal:Daily Fitness Goal:** Give your body some needed rest from a high-intensity workout. You can opt to work in an active yoga stretch such as "Refresh, Relax, and Restore: Stretching, Pilates, Yoga Workout for Tight Muscles" (youtube.com/watch?v= Pp8UNgkcAYs ), but don't forget to walk your 10,000 steps today!

## Breakfast

Most of us are in a rush in the morning. Here's an excellent way to create a delicious parfait with simple ingredients that are quick to prepare and that you can grab n' go!

• 6 ounces plain Greek yogurt layered with ¼ cup **Coconut Granola** and ½ cup sliced peaches

## Snack

• 1 tbsp. almond butter with 2 or more celery stalks

## Lunch

• 1 cup unsweetened fennel tea, hot or iced
• 4 ounces **Tuna-Avocado** and a large green salad that includes ½ cup cubed cooked or raw beets
• Recommended dressing pairing: 2 tbsp. **Miso Dressing**

## Snack

• 1 Health Warrior Chia Bar

## Dinner

• 1 cup unsweetened fennel tea, hot or iced
• 4 ounces **Kale Pesto Salmon** with 1 cup **Spicy Edamame in Pods** and **Roasted Turmeric Cauliflower**

## ⊶ BETH'S PREP TIPS

- Store the granola in airtight bag or container. You will be using another ¼ cup on Day 20.
- If you opt not to eat anything processed, simply substitute any bar on the plan for a veggie-based snack and protein (except for nuts) from the Meal Exchange List.
- You will have Kale Pesto Sauce again on Day 9. If you didn't prepare it in advance, freeze leftovers in 2 tbsp. servings in an ice cube tray.

# Day Three Recipes

## COCONUT GRANOLA

Yield: 24 servings

### Ingredients

1 cup pecans, chopped
1 cup raw cashews, chopped
1 cup raw slivered almonds
1 cup unsweetened shredded coconut
1 egg white, lightly beaten with 2 tbsp. water
3 tbsp. walnut oil
⅓ cup agave or maple syrup
1 tsp. vanilla extract
1 tsp. ground cinnamon
¼ tsp. Kosher salt
1 cup dried cranberries and/or dark chocolate chips, optional

### Directions

1. Preheat the oven to 300°F.
2. Place all ingredients into a medium-sized mixing bowl.
3. Stir to combine thoroughly.
4. Spread the granola on a large baking sheet lined with parchment paper. Be careful to spread the granola *evenly* and not stack it on top of each other.
5. Bake about 30 minutes, but be sure to mix it every 10 minutes. Watch it to ensure it doesn't burn and evenly bakes!
6. Let the granola cool at least 10 minutes so it can harden. Break into "clumps."

*Per serving (¼ cup) without optional ingredients: 140 calories, 12g fat, 3g saturated fat, 0mg cholesterol, 25mg sodium, 8g carbohydrate, 2g fiber, 3g protein*

## TUNA-AVOCADO

Yield: 1 serving

### Ingredients

1 (5-ounce) can light tuna
¼ ripe avocado
Suggested additions: finely chopped carrots, peppers, and/or celery
Garlic powder, salt, and pepper, to taste

### Directions

1. In a medium bowl, mash the tuna and avocado together.
2. Add any vegetables you desire to the tuna-avocado mixture.
3. Season with garlic powder, salt, and pepper, to taste.

*Per serving: 270 calories, 9g fat, 1.5g saturated fat, 50mg cholesterol, 85mg sodium, 4g carbohydrates, 3g fiber, 43g protein*

## KALE PESTO SAUCE

Yield: 12 servings

### Ingredients

¼ cup pine nuts
2 cups fresh kale, firmly packed
3 garlic cloves
1 tsp. sea salt
2 tbsp. extra-virgin olive oil

### Directions

1. Preheat the oven to 400°F.
2. Place the pine nuts on a baking sheet lined with parchment paper and toast until golden, about 3 minutes.
3. Place the kale in a food processor, add the pine nuts, garlic, and salt. Pulse until the kale is finely chopped.
4. Drizzle in the olive oil and continue to pulse until the pesto sauce reaches the desired consistency.

*Per serving (1 tbsp.): 48 calories, 4g fat, 0g saturated fat, 0mg cholesterol, 203mg sodium, 2g carbohydrates, 1g fiber, 1g protein*

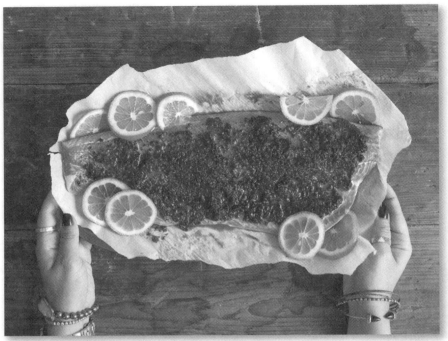

*For a color photo, see page 177.*

## KALE PESTO SALMON

Yield: 4 servings

### Ingredients

1 pound wild salmon, with skin
½ lemon
¼ cup (about 4 tbsp.) **Kale Pesto Sauce**

### Directions

1. Preheat the oven to 350°F.
2. Line a baking tray with parchment paper.
3. Lay the fish, skin side down, on the parchment paper.
4. Squeeze the lemon over the fish.
5. Spread the pesto sauce to cover the top and sides of the fish.
6. Bake about 10 minutes, then broil for 5 more minutes.

*Per serving: 232 calories, 14g fat, 3g saturated fat, 53mg cholesterol, 130mg sodium, 2g carbohydrates, 1g fiber, 23g protein*

## SPICY EDAMAME

Yield: 2 servings

### Ingredients

1 (1-pound) bag frozen or fresh edamame in the pod (green soybeans)
1 tsp. sea salt
1 tsp. chili powder
¼ to ½ tsp. red pepper flakes, to taste
½ tsp. oregano

### Directions

1. Boil the edamame pods in salted water about 8 minutes.
2. Drain the pods and let them dry.
3. Toss the edamame with the chili powder, oregano, and red paper flakes.
4. This dish is best served warm.

*Per serving: 120 calories, 5g fat, 1g saturated fat, 0mg cholesterol, 607mg sodium, 10g carbohydrates, 5g fiber, 10g protein*

## ROASTED TURMERIC CAULIFLOWER

Yield: 4 servings

### Ingredients

1 head cauliflower, separated into florets or 1 (32-ounce) bag frozen cauliflower, thawed and drained
1 tbsp. coconut oil, melted
1 tsp. turmeric
½ tsp. ground cumin
½ tsp. crushed red pepper flakes
½ tsp. crushed garlic

### Directions

1. Preheat the oven to 400°F.
2. Whisk together the coconut oil, turmeric, cumin, red pepper, and garlic.
3. Place the cauliflower on a baking sheet and coat with the spice mixture.
4. Roast the cauliflower for 30 minutes.

*Per serving: 45 calories, 2.5g fat, 2g saturated fat, 0mg cholesterol, 30mg sodium, 5g carbohydrates, 2g fiber, 2g protein*

# DAY FOUR

## Mindful Meditation to Start Your Day

*"Rabbi Meir used to say: Do not look at the flask but at what is in it; there may be a new flask that is full of old wine and an old flask that does not even have new wine in it."*

—ETHICS OF THE FATHERS 4:27

It's always easier to judge and compare ourselves to others by what is evident outside instead of what may be going on inside. I often hear frustration from clients who cannot understand why someone who may be the same age, gender, and height could lose weight faster than themselves. However, surface observations should not be the focus because it is not telling the full story. Perhaps the other people are struggling with stress, feeling sick, or exercising multiple times per day. Although they may look thin, they may have a high proportion of fat inside their body. It could be that they are super strict with their daily diets whereas you may be allowing yourself certain flexibilities. Other times, they may be losing at a faster rate simply because it works for their own body and does not necessarily mean there is anything wrong with them or you or that they are doing something different.

Research cannot predict why some people of the same measurements lose weight faster or reach a plateau quicker than another person. Ultimately, we need to believe that as long as we are doing the most we can for our diets and health, we are losing weight at the pace and amount that is right for our *own* bodies. You will be more likely to sustain weight loss when working *with* your body instead of a continuously shocking and working *against* it.

No one is like you. Therefore, you will not lose weight the same as someone else. Once you accept this, you can begin to look inside yourself and connect internally to what is unique about you. Take a deeper intuitive peak today by discovering the great things about you that can spread onto others. You may have a character trait of kindness, being a good friend, or the gift of making people smile; whatever it is, focus on what's inside your flask and show it to the world.

## For Starters

 **Kosher Cleanse Elixir:** Drink upon waking (see page 97).

 **Daily Fitness Goal:** Aside from your daily 10,000 steps today, begin to fall deeper into a yoga flow with this 50-minute routine (youtu.be/ lwprTau7-go).

## Breakfast

• **Kale Avocado Smoothie**

## Snack

• **KIND Bar** variety with less than 5g sugar

## Lunch

• 1 cup unsweetened green tea, hot or iced
• ½ avocado, mashed with juice of ½ lemon, cumin, and red pepper flakes on 1 slice sprouted grain bread, toasted, and **Tomato Salad**

## Snack

• 2 tbsp. hummus with 2 or more cucumbers

## Dinner

• 1 cup unsweetened fennel tea, hot or iced
• **Collard Wraps with Turkey Meatballs, Avocado, and Dijon** and 1 small baked potato with skin

## ♡ BETH'S PREP TIPS

- Add 1 cup of ice to make the smoothie colder if using fresh produce.
- Serve 3 meatballs with tonight's dinner, then cool the remaining meatballs completely before storing them in an airtight container in the fridge.
- Be sure to freeze the leftover ground turkey for Days 8 and 10.
- Don't forget to prep your **Chia Yogurt** recipe and store it in the refrigerator for tomorrow's breakfast!

# Day Four Recipes

## KALE AVOCADO SMOOTHIE

Yield: 1 serving

### Ingredients

½ avocado
½ cup kale
½ cup frozen cauliflower florets
½ cup low-fat plain Greek yogurt
1 cup unsweetened vanilla almond milk
1/4 cup frozen mango chunks

### Directions

Put all ingredients in Vitamix or blender. Blend on high for 30 seconds until creamy.

*Per serving: 340 calories, 18g fat, 2.5g saturated fat, 280mg sodium, 10mg cholesterol, 7g carbohydrates, 11g fiber, 23g protein*

## TOMATO SALAD

Yield: 1 serving

### Ingredients

1 (10.5-ounce) container multicolored cherry tomatoes, halved
Juice of 1 lemon
¼ tsp. salt
Dash of white pepper
2 tsp. extra-virgin olive oil
2 cloves garlic, minced

### Directions

1. Combine all ingredients in medium mixing bowl.
2. Adjust the seasonings to taste.

*Per serving: 132 calories, 9g fat, 1.5g saturated fat, 580mg sodium, 0g cholesterol, 11g carbohydrates, 3g fiber, 2g protein*

## COLLARD WRAPS WITH TURKEY MEATBALLS, AVOCADO, AND DIJON

Yield: 1 serving

### Ingredients

3 large collard green leaves,
   washed, dried, stems removed

Sea salt

3 **Big Batch Turkey Meatballs**

¼ avocado, thinly sliced

1 large beefsteak tomato,
   thinly sliced

2 tsp. Dijon mustard

### Directions

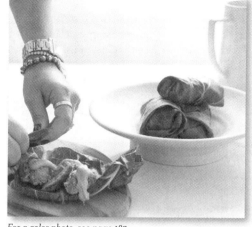

*For a color photo, see page 183.*

1. Put the collard greens into a large saucepan with 1 cup of cold water. Bring the water to a boil, add a pinch of sea salt, and cover. Reduce the heat and cook until the leaves are wilted and just tender, about 5 to 10 minutes depending on the size and toughness of the leaves.
2. Lay the collard greens flat on a cutting board, and top with one turkey meatball.
3. Mash each meatball with a fork until it's about ¼-inch thick.
4. Top each smashed meatball with equal amounts of avocado and tomato with a dollop of mustard.
5. Roll up each leaf and transfer to a plate to serve.

*Per serving (based on 4 ounces of turkey): 300 calories, 17g fat, 3.5g saturated fat, 70mg cholesterol, 24g carbohydrates, 235mg sodium, 9g fiber, 16g protein*

## BIG BATCH TURKEY MEATBALLS

Yield: 24

### Ingredients

⅓ cup rolled oats, ground into a flour in a Vitamix or blender, pulsed until the consistency of breadcrumbs

½ onion, chopped

1 egg

1 lb. chopped turkey

4 basil leaves, chopped

¼ tsp. Kosher salt

¼ tsp. chili powder

Dash of freshly ground pepper

*(recipe continues, page 120)*

## Directions

1. Preheat the oven to 400°F.
2. Line a small rimmed baking sheet with parchment paper (if you only have a large sheet you can use that instead).
3. Combine the oats, onion, egg, turkey, salt, chili powder, and pepper in a medium mixing bowl, and mix everything with a rubber spatula until the mixture is combined and uniform throughout.
4. Form the turkey mixture into 6 balls and space them apart on the baking sheet.
5. Bake 15 minutes or until the meatballs are cooked through (there should be no pink inside, and a thermometer inserted into the center of a meatball should read 165°F).

*Per serving (3 meatballs): 170 calories, 9g fat, 2.5g saturated fat, 105mg sodium, 70mg cholesterol, 10g carbohydrates, 2g fiber, 12g protein*

(Source: BuzzFeedFood.com)

# DAY FIVE

# SABBATH NIGHT

## Mindful Meditation to Start Your Day

*"As long as the candle is still burning, it is still possible to accomplish and to mend."*

—RABBI YISRAEL SALANTER (1809-1883), FATHER OF THE MUSAR (MORAL CONDUCT) MOVEMENT IN ORTHODOX JUDAISM AND A FAMED ROSH YESHIVA (HEAD OF RELIGIOUS EDUCATION) AND TALMUDIST

*One night, Rabbi Salanter was walking home past the home of a shoemaker. Despite it being very late, he observed the shoemaker was still busy, working by the light of a single candle. "Why are you still working?" Rabbi Salanter asked him. "It is very late, and soon the candle will go out."*

*The shoemaker replied, "As long as the candle is still burning it is still possible to accomplish and to mend shoes." In his wisdom, Rabbi Salanter realized this message is true for all of us. It's never too late to change.\**

---

\* Miller, Y. (2016, September 24). *Inspiring Jewish Quotes for Rosh Hashana*. Retrieved on September 3, 2017 from aish.com/sp/pg/Inspiring-Jewish-Quotes-for-Rosh-Hashanah.html

It sometimes feels like we can never change because we are stuck in our ways. We may continue to engage in bad habits simply because it's something we have always done. Well, that excuse stops now. I too often see people accepting harmful habits because they feel defeated. They think they are incapable of changing and wallow in their weak moments. Going into the weekend is another potential area to succumb to diet weaknesses. Don't let the shadows of your poor old habits consume you. Remember, we talked about how any life struggle is put into our path for a reason and is meant for us to overcome so that we can grow. It may take blood, sweat, and tears, but know that you can and will change. Keep up your hard work, you are earning these results, and because of that, they will feel more meaningful!

##  BETH'S PREP TIPS

It's Friday! You may want to go grocery shopping for week 2 so you can start prepping on Sunday for the week ahead.

## For Starters

 **Kosher Cleanse Elixir:** Drink upon waking (see page 97).

 **Daily Fitness Goal:** Aside from walking your 10,000 steps today, get ready for the weekend with another HIIT workout to get you burning fat, "Furious Fat Burner 2" Home HIIT Cardio Workout / Burn Fat Fast (youtube.com/watch?v=jr6DuNMTQBc). Feeling strong? Try it twice or combine it with a yoga stretch.

## Breakfast

• 1 cup **Chia Yogurt** with ½ cup blueberries and sliced strawberries

## Snack

• 12 cherries with 8 walnut halves

# Lunch

- 1 cup unsweetened green tea, hot or iced ☕
- 2 **Gal's Black Bean Burger** on a large salad filled with non-starchy veggies
- Recommended dressing pairing: 2 tbsp. **Miso Dressing**

# Snack

- 3 tbsp. **Guacamole** and 1 or more red, yellow, and/or orange bell pepper

# Dinner

For Friday night dinner and Saturday lunch, or the "Sabbath" meals in Judaism, it is an obligation to make a blessing over bread (or "challah") and red wine as well as a custom to consume red meat. In order to hold true to the tradition of a kosher girl's diet, and thanks to the help of recipe developing with my strategist, Sarah Kassin, and her Harari family, I worked in the unique foods and beverages that align with my nutrition strategy so that you do not fall off the plan. Instead you'll feel as if your weekend meals are festive. Regardless of whether you keep the Sabbath or not, the opportunity to consume a mindful meal and food options that are different than the rest of the week will help keep you feeling excited about sticking with your whole foods on the plan and teach you how to incorporate a more realistic way of eating that you can maintain beyond the 21 days.

- 1 cup unsweetened fennel tea, hot or iced ☕
- 4 ounces red wine (counts as an after-dinner optional snack if this is your Sabbath night meal)
- 3 ounces **organic grass-fed Brisket** with ½ cup **Wild Rice,** cooked (or the "challah" whole wheat sourdough bread, if mandatory)

## 🫀 BETH'S PREP TIPS

- If you want to avoid red meat, use 4 ounces of any chicken or fish recipe.
- Roast the **Japanese Sweet Potatoes**, cook the **Kale Chips**, and grill the chicken breast today so that they can be ready for lunch tomorrow.

# Day Five Recipes

## CHIA YOGURT

Yield: 1 serving

### Ingredients

¼ cup chia seeds
1 cup unsweetened almond milk, homemade or store-bought
1 tsp. vanilla extract
¼ tsp. ground cinnamon, optional
½ cup blueberries and sliced strawberries, optional

### Directions

1. Whisk the chia seeds, almond milk, vanilla, cinnamon and berries, if desired, in a Mason jar or container.
2. Refrigerate at least 4 hours or overnight to form a gel-like consistency.

*Per serving (with berries): 310 calories, 17g fat, 1.5g saturated fat, 0mg cholesterol, 190mg sodium, 32g carbohydrates, 18g fiber, 9g protein*

## GAL'S BLACK BEAN BURGERS

Gal Shua-Haim (founder of the Instagram account @holyhealth and Beth Warren Nutrition dietitian) created these veggie burgers and served them on our first Kosher Cleanse retreat. They were such a huge hit that I had to share her recipe!

Yield: 6 servings

### Ingredients

⅓ white onion, grated
1 (15-ounce) can black beans, rinsed, drained, and mashed
½ cup oat flour (¾ cup oats ground into flour)
⅓ cup parsley
1 tbsp. tomato paste
2 to 3 tsp. Cajun seasoning (based on taste preference)
1 tbsp. ground flax seed
1 tsp. salt
½ tsp. pepper

### Directions

1. Preheat the oven to 350°F.
2. Combine all the ingredients in a large bowl.
3. Form into patties to make 6 regular-sized burgers.
4. Bake about 8 minutes on each side.

*Per serving: 100 calories, 1.5g fat, 0g saturated fat, 0mg cholesterol, 850mg sodium, 17g carbs, 5g fiber, 5g protein*

## BRISKET

Yield: 8 servings

### Ingredients

2½ lb. brisket
*For the sauce:*
1 small onion, chopped
2 cloves garlic, minced
1 tbsp. extra-virgin olive oil, plus
    more for sautéing
½ cup tomato sauce
¼ cup prune juice
1 tsp. honey
1 tsp. molasses
⅛ cup red wine vinegar
⅛ cup cooking wine
1 tsp. garlic powder
½ tsp. salt
1 tsp. mustard

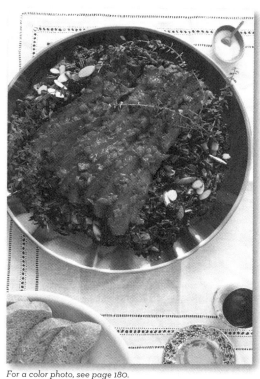

*For a color photo, see page 180.*

### Directions

1. Preheat the oven to 350°F.
2. Sauté the onion and garlic in olive oil in a deep pan over medium heat.
3. Put the brisket in the pan and brown on all sides, flipping the roast over as needed.
4. In a bowl, combine the tomato sauce, prune juice, honey, molasses, vinegar, wine, garlic powder, salt, mustard and the 1 tbsp. oil.
5. Put half the sauce in the roast pan and bake for 1 hour, covered.
6. Transfer the brisket to a roaster and pour the sauce over the brisket, reserving a small amount for serving.
7. Bake 1 more hour.
8. Cool, then slice.

*Per serving: 341 calories, 16g fat, 5g saturated fat, 132mg cholesterol, 223mg sodium, 4g carbohydrates, <1g fiber, 43g protein*

## WILD RICE

Yield: 6 servings

### Ingredients

1 onion, chopped
1 tbsp. extra-virgin olive oil
1 cup wild rice
2 cups low-sodium organic vegetable broth
Salt and pepper, to taste
¼ cup sliced almonds
1/8 cup dried cherries (no sugar added), chopped

### Directions

1. In a medium saucepan, sauté the onion in the oil until softened.
2. Add the wild rice and broth.
3. Season with salt and pepper, adjust to low heat, and cover.
4. Cook about 20 minutes and remove the pan from the burner.
5. Fold in the almonds and cherries.

*Per serving (½ cup): 160 calories, 4.5g fat, 0.5g saturated fat, 320mg sodium, 0mg cholesterol, 26g carbohydrates, 3g fiber, 5g protein*

## GARLIC MUSTARD STRING BEANS

Yield: 2 servings

### Ingredients

1 lb. frozen French-style string beans
1 tbsp. extra-virgin olive oil
4 tbsp. Dijon mustard
4 cloves garlic, minced

### Directions

1. Preheat the oven to 400°F.
2. Line a baking sheet with parchment paper and put the string beans on the pan.
3. Mix together the olive oil, mustard, and garlic; rub onto the string beans.
4. Bake 20 minutes or until the beans reach the desired crispness.

*Per serving: 127 calories, 7g fat, 7.5g fat, 402mg sodium, 7.5g carbohydrates, 4g fiber, 1.5g protein*

# DAY SIX

# SABBATH DAY

## Mindful Meditation to Start Your Day

*"If you are not going to be better tomorrow than you were today, then what need have you for tomorrow?"*

—REBBE NACHMAN OF BRESLOV

Each of us faces challenges daily. We also have a choice in how we react to these struggles. The easy way out is to give up; however, the only way to improve and grow is to wake up the next day and make a choice to continue onward. The weekends present temptations that are hard to overcome. It may seem like a lose-lose situation because if we veer off the diet a bit then we feel guilty and if we keep the diet too strictly then we feel sad to miss out on indulgences. Dwelling on these negative feelings will only sabotage your efforts in sticking to a plan.

Choose to grasp the new opportunities another day presents. Each morning, push yourself towards recommitting and refocusing yourself on your goals. You have the potential to work through any challenge that pops up while following the diet and come out stronger. Always aim to reach higher than where you are now. You can always improve. Aim to be better, not perfect. You can do this.

## For Starters

 **Kosher Cleanse Elixir:** Drink upon waking (see page 97).

 **Daily Fitness Goal:** The Sabbath is known as a day of rest, and resting is literally what you will be doing. Remember, resting means you can still get your walking in or do light yoga stretches.

## Breakfast

- 2 **Oat Apple Muffins**

## Snack

- 3 fresh apricots with ½ ounces shelled raw pumpkin seeds

## Lunch

- 1 cup unsweetened green tea, hot or iced
- 4 ounces (for women) 6 ounces (for men) chicken breast and **large salad** with choice of dressing and **In a Jiffy Bean Salad**. (Skip the Bean Salad if you choose the 2 ounces whole wheat sourdough slice.)

## Snack

- 2 cups **Kale Chips** with 1 tbsp. nutritional yeast

## Dinner

- 1 cup unsweetened fennel tea, hot or iced
- **Spanish Omelet** with a side of 1 cup freshly popped organic popcorn

 **BETH'S PREP TIPS**

- Store the **Kale Chips** in a brown bag and make enough to be used as a snack for Day 16.
- Freeze the leftover **In a Jiffy Bean Salad** in ½-cup-sized portions to be eaten again on Day 10 dinner and Day 19 snack.

# Day Six Recipes

## OAT APPLE MUFFINS

Yield: 12

### Ingredients

2 eggs
1 cup Greek yogurt
⅓ cup coconut sugar
2 tsp. vanilla extract
2½ cups rolled oats
2 tsp. baking powder
Pinch of salt
1 tbsp. ground cinnamon
2 apples, peeled, cored, and grated
1 cup unsweetened almond milk

### Directions

1. Preheat the oven to 350°F.
2. In a large bowl, beat the eggs with a whisk until they are foamy and pale yellow.
3. Add the Greek yogurt, coconut sugar, and vanilla to the bowl; whisk until the mixture thickens and is well combined (it will still be a little runny).
4. Sprinkle the oats, baking powder, salt, cinnamon, and apple over the egg mixture.
5. Use a spatula to fold the wet and dry ingredients together.
6. Pour in the almond milk and continue mixing until everything is well incorporated (it will be a loose mixture).
7. Using a medium-sized ice cream scoop, scoop the batter into 12 muffin tin cups lined with cupcake liners. Fill cups close to the top as these muffins do not rise too high.
8. Bake 35 to 40 minutes, until the muffins have set and just started to turn golden brown.

*Per serving (2 muffins): 220 calories, 4.5g fat, 1g saturated fat, 35mg cholesterol, 40mg sodium, 36g carbohydrates, 4g fiber, 9g protein*

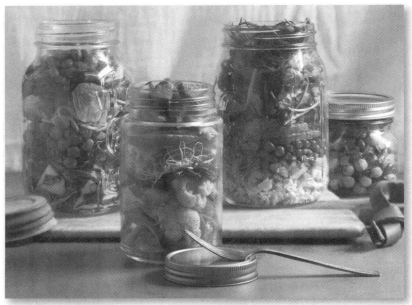

*For a color photo, see page 181.*

## IN A JIFFY BEAN SALAD

Yield: 6 servings

### Ingredients

1 (15-ounce) can no-salt or reduced sodium red kidney beans, rinsed
1 (15-ounce) can no-salt or reduced sodium black beans, rinsed
1 (15-ounce) can no-salt or reduced sodium chickpeas, rinsed
1 medium red onion, diced small
1 red pepper, seeded and diced small
½ cup chopped fresh parsley
1/3 cup apple cider vinegar
1/3 cup fresh lemon juice
2/3 cup extra-virgin olive oil
1 tsp. Himalayan sea salt
Black pepper, to taste

### Directions

Combine all ingredients in a large bowl, and serve. You can refrigerate the salad up to 5 days.

*Per serving: 346 calories, 25g fat, 3g saturated fat, m mg cholesterol, 391mg sodium, 26g carbohydrates, 7g fiber, 8g protein*

(Recipe by: Healthful Pursuits)

## KALE CHIPS

### Ingredients

Kale, 1 head, separates into leaves and chopped
Salt and pepper, to taste
Desired seasonings such as zaatar, optional

### Directions

1. Preheat the oven to 350°F.
2. Place the kale on a baking sheet in a single layer.
3. Sprinkle with salt and pepper and any other desired seasoning, to taste.
4. Place into the oven and leave the oven door slightly ajar. Bake about 10 minutes. Keep checking on the kale chips so they do not burn.

## SPANISH OMELET

Yield: 1 serving

### Ingredients

3 egg whites plus 1 egg yolk
1 cup onion, sliced thinly and vertically
4 garlic cloves, minced
2 tbsp. chopped fresh oregano, divided
¾ tsp. Kosher salt
¼ tsp. freshly ground black pepper
Spritz of nonstick cooking spray

### Directions

1. Mix eggs in a bowl with the onion, garlic, oregano, salt, and pepper.
2. Pour the egg mixture into a pan that's been sprayed with the nonstick cooking spray. Cook on medium heat until the omelet edges are crispy. Then flip over to cook the other side.

*Per serving: 224 calories, 5g fat, 2g saturated fat, 186mg cholesterol, 750mg sodium, 18g carbohydrates, 3g fiber, 16g protein*

# DAY SEVEN

## Mindful Meditation to Start Your Day

*"The entire purpose of our existence is to overcome our negative habits."*

—VILNA GAON, COMMENTARY TO MISHLEI 4:13

You are on a one-way track heading towards eliminating harmful habits that you may not have known you had a week ago. Although after a weekend, a time that's hard foodwise for anyone regardless of religion, age, or gender, you probably recognized a few common temptations. Each day you are creating positive changes that will form into new habits at the completion of the diet. Don't get nervous from symptoms and feelings that may creep up as the early days pass. You're trans-forming your status quo of living and eating, which is bound to bring up a lot of emotional and physical changes. Simply jot down your progress in the Wellness Planner. By recording your thoughts throughout the diet, you can figure out which types of food and lifestyle factors are working for you. Trust me: You will reach a point where the efforts will feel more natural and your overall mood and energy will improve. Stick with it!

 **BETH'S PREP TIPS**

It's Sunday! Be sure to prepare your snacks for the week!

# For Starters

 **Kosher Cleanse Elixir:** Drink upon waking (see page 97).

 **Daily Fitness Goal:** Jump into the upcoming week with a powerful workout. Try this one: TABATA Workout for Fat Burning & Toning / HIIT Workout No Equipment. (youtube.com/watch?v=nKIU42Z51tU) Don't forget to walk your 10,000 steps today!

# Breakfast

• **Detox Protein Smoothie**

# Snack

• ¼ mango with 23 raw pistachios

# Lunch

• Tuna (one 4-ounce can) on a large salad with lots of non-starchy veggies with ½ cup peas (I recommend raw frozen peas) plus 10 Mary's Gone Crackers.

• Recommended dressing pairing: 2 tbsp. **Balsamic Dressing**

# Snack

• 1 (6-ounce) container of grass-fed plain Greek yogurt with ½ cup blueberries

# Dinner

• 2 cups **Lentil Soup** and **Turmeric Cauliflower**

 **BETH'S PREP TIPS**

Freeze the leftover Lentil Soup to be eaten again on Day 18.

# Day Seven Recipes

## DETOX PROTEIN SMOOTHIE

Yield: 1 serving

### Ingredients

2 handfuls baby spinach, rinsed
1 tsp. freshly grated ginger
2 cups frozen sliced peaches
1¼ cup water
2 scoops grass-fed whey protein powder

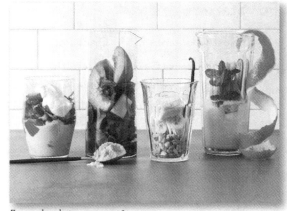

*For a color photo, see page 182.*

### Directions

1. Cut off a thumb tip-sized piece of ginger and pulse in a blender to grate it.
2. Add the spinach, peaches, water, and protein power; blend until smooth.

*Per serving: 135 calories, 0g fat, 0g saturated fat, 0g cholesterol, 210mg sodium, 13g carbohydrates, 2g fiber, 22g protein*

## TURMERIC CAULIFLOWER

Yield: 4 servings

### Ingredients

1 tbsp. coconut oil, melted
1 tsp. turmeric
½ tsp. ground cumin
½ tsp. crushed red pepper
½ tsp. crushed garlic
1 head cauliflower, separated into florets

### Directions

1. Preheat the oven to 400°F.
2. Whisk together the coconut oil, turmeric, cumin, red pepper, and garlic.
3. Place the cauliflower florets on a sheet pan and coat with the coconut oil-spice mixture.
4. Roast the cauliflower for 30 minutes.

*Per serving: 45 calories, 2.5g fat, 2g saturated fat, 0mg cholesterol, 30mg sodium, 5g carbohydrates, 2g fiber, 2g protein*

## LENTIL SOUP

Yield: 4 servings

### Ingredients

1 cup split red lentils, rinsed
4 cups water
2 large cloves garlic, crushed
½ tsp. coriander
1 tbsp. coarse salt
2 tbsp. extra-virgin olive oil
Ground cumin and crushed red pepper, to taste
Lemon juice, to taste, optional

### Directions

1. Add the lentils to the water in a medium-sized saucepan
2. Bring to a boil over low heat, until the lentils are creamy. Remove from the heat.
3. In a medium-sized pan, sauté the garlic, coriander, and salt in the olive oil.
4. Add the garlic mixture to the lentils, return the pan to low heat, and simmer for 1 hour.
5. Serve with a pinch of cumin, crushed red pepper, and lemon juice, if desired.

*Per serving: 210 calories, 7g fat, 0.5g saturated fat, 0mg cholesterol, 365mg sodium, 28g carbohydrates, 7g fiber, 11g protein*

# DAY EIGHT

## Mindful Meditation to Start Your Day

*"Examine the contents, not the bottle."*

—ETHICS OF OUR FATHERS 4:27

The time has come for your weigh-in. It's common to feel anxious; however, it is ultimately what is inside that counts, not what is outside. Today, the thought is cliché; however, the quoted Talmudic reference inferred it ages ago. It's important to remind yourself to always look inside at the forefront of your mind. How you view yourself physically can be misleading and does not always reflect accurately in the number on the scale. Your weight is a small factor in the scope of your diet success, which is one reason why you should not give the scale power over your mood. Use the weigh-in as a check-in with yourself, note it on your Wellness Planner, and keep moving forward!

## For Starters

 **Kosher Cleanse Elixir:** Drink upon waking (see page 97).

 **Daily Fitness Goal:** Work in your choice of yoga routine today that focuses on various body parts you want to target, for example, *Yoga for Abs and Arms Workout with Caitlin Turner*. Keep up with getting in your 10,000 steps today!

## Breakfast

• **Spinach Mushroom Omelet** with 1 cup cubed melon

# Snack

- **Mixed Nuts:** 1 (100-calorie pack) with non-starchy veggies or ½ ounce any raw nut combo (8 walnuts, 10 cashews, or 10 pecans)

# Lunch

- **Vegetarian Chili with Quinoa** (2 cups) plus a large salad filled with non-starchy veggies and 2 tbsp. of any choice of dressing

# Snack

- **Health Warrior Chia Bar** (1 bar)

# Dinner

- 1 cup unsweetened fennel tea, hot or iced
- **Turkey Meat Sauce** and **Tomato Zoodles** (4 ounces)
- **Butternut Squash Soup**, 1 cup (See Beth Tip)

## BETH'S PREP TIPS

- You can purchase the store-bought packs of 100-calorie **unsalted nut mixes**.
- Freeze the extra **Butternut Squash Soup** to eat on Day 10.
- Prep the **Chia Yogurt** for tomorrow's breakfast.

# Day Eight Recipes

## SPINACH MUSHROOM OMELET

Yield: 1 omelet

### Ingredients

3 egg whites plus 1 egg yolk, whisked
nonstick cooking spray
¼ cup chopped shallots
1 garlic clove, minced
¼ cup sliced white mushrooms
1 sprig thyme
2 ounces fresh baby spinach, rinsed
¼ tsp. Kosher salt
⅛ tsp. freshly ground black pepper

### Directions

1. Heat a medium-sized cast-iron skillet on medium heat sprayed with nonstick cooking spray.
2. Add the shallots, garlic, mushrooms, and thyme.
3. Sauté 7 minutes or until the mushrooms are browned.
4. Add the spinach and sauté 4 minutes, or until the liquid almost evaporates.
5. Remove the mixture from the skillet; discard the thyme.
6. Add the eggs to pan for one minute and then add vegetables, salt and pepper. Flip when the omelet starts to crisp.

*Per serving: serves 1: 146 calories, 5g fat, 2g saturated fat, 350mg sodium, 186mg cholesterol, 10g carbohydrates, .7g fiber, 16g protein*

## VEGETARIAN CHILI WITH QUINOA

Yields: 10 to 12 servings. (This chili freezes well.)

### Ingredients

½ cup quinoa, rinsed
1 cup water
1 tbsp. extra-virgin olive oil
1 small onion, chopped
3 cloves garlic, minced
1 jalapeño pepper, seeded and diced
1 large carrot, peeled and chopped
2 celery stalks, chopped
1 green bell pepper, seeded and chopped
1 red bell pepper, seeded and chopped
1 medium zucchini, chopped

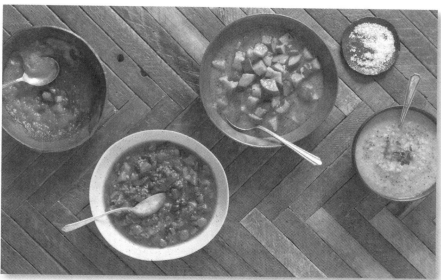

*For a color photo, see page 176.*

2 (15-ounce) cans black beans, drained and rinsed
1 (15-ounce) can red kidney beans, drained and rinsed
3 (15-ounce) cans diced tomatoes
1 (15-ounce) can tomato sauce
2 to 3 tbsp. chili powder, depending on your taste preference
1 tbsp. ground cumin
Salt and black pepper, to taste

### Directions

1. In a medium saucepan, combine the quinoa and water.
2. Cook over medium heat until the water is absorbed, about 15 minutes. Set aside.
3. In a large pot, heat the olive oil over high heat.
4. Add the onion and cook until tender, about 5 minutes.
5. Stir in garlic, jalapeño, carrot, celery, bell peppers, and zucchini.
6. Cook until the vegetables are tender, about 10 minutes.
7. Add the black beans, kidney beans, tomatoes, and tomato sauce. Stir in the cooked quinoa.
8. Season with the chili powder, cumin, salt, and pepper.
9. Simmer the chili on low about 30 minutes. Serve warm.

(Adapted from: twopeasandtheirpod.com)

## TURKEY MEAT SAUCE

Yields: 8 servings

### Ingredients

2 shallots or 1 onion, chopped
1 tbsp. extra-virgin olive oil
2 lbs. ground turkey
1 (15-ounce) can tomato sauce
½ cup no-sodium vegetable broth
1 tsp. each of cumin, sea salt, black pepper, dried oregano, crushed red pepper flakes

### Directions

1. In a large skillet over medium-high heat, sauté the shallots or onion in the olive oil until translucent.
2. Add the turkey. Cook, separating and turning it, until it's no longer pink, about 6 minutes.
3. Add the tomato sauce, broth, and the cumin, salt, black pepper, oregano, and red pepper.
4. Cover and simmer about 20 minutes.

*Per serving (4 ounces): 230 calories, 16g fat, 4g saturated fat, 540mg sodium, 90mg cholesterol, 3g carbohydrates, 1g fiber, 20g protein*

## TOMATO ZOODLES

Yields: 6 servings

### Ingredients

2 cloves garlic, crushed
1 tsp. extra-virgin olive oil
1 (15-ounce) can tomato sauce
Basil, salt, black pepper
Crushed red pepper flakes, optional
4 medium zucchini, spiralized

### Directions

1. Sauté the garlic in the olive oil on low heat.
2. Add the tomato sauce, reduce the heat and let simmer to thicken.
3. Season with basil, salt, pepper, and crushed red pepper flakes, if desired.
4. Turn off heat and stir the zucchini into the sauce.
5. Allow to rest until it reaches the desired consistency; then serve immediately.

*Per serving: 56 calories, 1g fat, 0g saturated fat, 468mg sodium, 0mg cholesterol, 10g carbohydrates, 2g fiber, 2g protein*

## BUTTERNUT SQUASH SOUP

Yields: 6 servings

### Ingredients

3 pounds butternut squash (about 2 medium),
    cut in half lengthwise, seeds removed
Cooking spray
5 tsp. extra-virgin olive oil, divided
1 large onion, finely chopped
¼ cup chopped fresh parsley
2 tbsp. fresh or ½ tsp. dried sage
½ tsp. chopped fresh or ⅛ tsp. dried thyme
4½ cups water
1½ tsp. salt, divided
½ tsp. coarse black pepper, divided
2 garlic cloves, minced
1 tbsp. balsamic vinegar
2 cups radicchio, thinly sliced, divided

### Directions

1. Preheat the oven to 375°F.
2. Place the squash, cut sides down, on a foil-lined baking sheet coated with cooking spray.
3. Bake for 30 minutes or until tender. Scoop out the pulp; set aside. Discard the skins.
4. Heat 1 tbsp. oil in a large Dutch oven over medium heat. Add the onion, parsley, sage, and thyme; cook 15 minutes or until the onion is lightly browned, stirring frequently.
5. Add the squash, water, 1¼ tsp. salt, ¼ tsp. pepper, and garlic; bring to a boil.
6. Partially cover, reduce heat, and simmer 25 minutes. Place about 2½ cups of the squash mixture in a blender, and process until smooth. Pour the pureéd soup into a large bowl. Repeat procedure with remaining squash mixture, 2½ cups at a time.
7. Heat 1 tbsp. oil in a large nonstick skillet over medium-high heat. Add the radicchio, ¼ tsp. salt, and ¼ tsp. pepper. Sauté 5 minutes or until the radicchio is lightly browned.
8. Remove from heat and drizzle with the vinegar, tossing to coat. Ladle 1⅓ cups soup into each of 6 bowls. Top each serving with ⅓ cup radicchio.

*Per serving: 210 calories, 4.5g fat, 0.5g saturated fat, 610mg sodium, 0mg cholesterol, 43g carbohydrates, 8g fiber, 5g protein*

# DAY NINE

## Mindful Meditation to Start Your Day

*"A sudden transition from one opposite to another*
*is impossible and therefore man, according to his nature,*
*is not capable of abandoning suddenly all*
*to which he was accustomed."*

—RABBI MOSHE BEN MAIMON, GUIDE FOR THE PERPLEXED 3:23

It is possible for us to make significant changes in our lives, but
Maimonides' advice reminds us to take it slow, one step at a time.
Taking incremental steps makes it more likely that we stick with
new resolutions and routines.

I understand how frustrating it may seem to make small changes
incrementally over time. I can see the appeal of quick fixes and fad
diets that provide highly processed bars and shakes as your source
of sustenance for ease and convenience. Trust in the process that
these changes you are making on my plan are not only effective short
term, but will guarantee long term success. You are not only targeting
total weight, you are targeting fat loss, boost in muscle and improvements in mood, energy levels and quality of life. Quick and easy fixes
may provide a short term loss in one area, but my plan is providing
you with long term benefits in many areas. In other words, it is worth
it so keep on going!

## For Starters

 **Kosher Cleanse Elixir:** Drink upon waking (see page 97).

 **Daily Fitness Goal:** Ease into the diet with a boost of motivation and physical fitness from your fitness choice from the Resources for Fitness. Don't forget to walk your 10,000 steps today!

## Breakfast

• **Chia Yogurt** with ½ cup berries

## Snack

• 3 **Almond Date Balls**

## Lunch

• Sprouted Grain Wrap with ½ avocado, 4 tbsp. hummus, and 1 tsp. **Kale Pesto Sauce** with **Israeli Salad**

## Snack

• 2 tbsp. hummus with 2 or more Persian cucumbers

## Dinner

• 1 cup unsweetened fennel tea, hot or iced
• 4 ounces grilled **Honey Mustard Wild Salmon**, 2 cups **Lemon Artichokes**, and ½ **Sweet Potato Boat**

---

**BETH'S PREP TIPS**

• Prepare and refrigerate your **Overnight Oats** tonight for tomorrow's breakfast.
• Defrost one ½ cup serving of **In a Jiffy Bean Salad** and ½ cup of **Butternut Squash Soup** to eat with tomorrow's dinner.

# Day Nine Recipes

## CHIA YOGURT WITH MIXED BERRIES

Yield: 1 serving

### Ingredients

1 cup unsweetened almond milk (homemade or store-bought)
¼ tsp. vanilla extract
¼ tsp. ground cinnamon, optional
¼ cup chia seeds
½ cup mixed berries

### Directions

1. Mix the almond milk, vanilla, and cinnamon together.
2. Whisk in the chia seeds. Pour the mixture into a jar or other glass container and refrigerate at least 4 hours or overnight to let the it gel. Top with berries to serve.

*Per serving (with fruit): 310 calories, 17g fat, 1.5g saturated fat, 0mg cholesterol, 190mg sodium, 32g carbohydrates, 18g fiber, 9g protein*

## 3 ALMOND DATE BALLS

Yield: 20 date balls

### Ingredients

1 cup pitted dates
1 tsp. vanilla extract
1 cup raw almonds
½ cup almond butter
½ tsp. ground cinnamon
Kosher salt
Unsweetened shredded coconut (optional)

### Directions

1. Process the dates in a food processor with the vanilla until smooth.
2. Mix all other ingredients into the food processor bowl and pulse. The consistency should be like cookie dough.
3. Form the dough into 1-inch balls and roll in the coconut, if desired.
4. Store in the refrigerator or freezer in an airtight container.

*Per serving (2 balls): 110 calories, 6g fat, 0g sat fat, 0mg cholesterol, 5mg sodium 11g carbohydrates, 2g fiber, 2g protein*

## KALE PESTO

Yields: 12 servings

### Ingredients

½ cup pine nuts
2 cups fresh kale, firmly packed
3 garlic cloves
1 tsp. sea salt
2 tbsp. extra-virgin olive oil

### Directions

1. Place the pine nuts in a dry cast-iron skillet and heat on medium until golden brown, about 3 minutes on medium heat.
2. Next, place the kale in a food processor, add the pine nuts, garlic, and salt. Pulse until the kale is finely chopped.
3. Drizzle the olive oil over the kale mixture and continue to pulse until the pesto reaches the desired consistency.

*Per serving: 48 calories, 4g fat, 0g saturated fat, 0mg cholesterol, 203mg sodium, 2g carbohydrates, 1g fiber, 1g protein*

## ISRAELI SALAD

Yield: 1 serving

### Ingredients

½ red onion, finely chopped
1 bunch parsley, finely chopped
2 cucumbers, finely chopped
1 tomato, finely chopped
1 tsp. extra-virgin olive oil
2 garlic cloves, minced
Juice of 1 lemon
Salt and pepper, to taste
Cumin, to taste (optional)

### Directions

Mix the onion, parsley, cucumbers, and tomato in a bowl with the olive oil, garlic, lemon, salt, pepper, and cumin, if desired.

*Per serving: 230 calories, 6g fat, 1g saturated fat, 75mg sodium, 0mg cholesterol, 46g carbohydrates, 8g fiber, 9g protein*

## HONEY MUSTARD WILD SALMON

Yield: 1 serving

### Ingredients

4 ounces wild salmon
1 tbsp. Dijon mustard
1 tbsp. extra-virgin olive oil
1 tsp. honey
2 tsp. fresh lemon juice, optional

### Directions

1. Preheat the oven to 350°F.
2. Line an oven-proof dish with parchment paper and place the salmon on the parchment.
3. Mix the Dijon mustard, olive oil, and honey until well combined; spread on the salmon.
4. Bake for 12 minutes.
5. Squeeze fresh lemon over the salmon before serving, if desired.

*Per serving: 190 calories, 8g fat, 1g saturated fat, 60 mg cholesterol, 210mg sodium, 7g carbohydrates, 1g fiber, 23g protein*

## SWEET POTATO BOAT

Yields: 6 servings

### Ingredients

3 medium-sized sweet potatoes
¼ small red onion, chopped
½ jalapeño, chopped, optional based on taste preference
1 tsp. avocado oil
1 cup crimini mushrooms, sliced
¼ tsp. ground cumin
¼ tsp. hot or sweet paprika
Sea salt and black pepper, to taste
Parsley for garnish (optional)

### Directions

1. Preheat the oven to 400°F.
2. Bake the sweet potatoes about 40 minutes or until tender.
3. Cut the sweet potatoes in half once they've been removed from the oven; set aside and allow to cool.
4. In a skillet, sauté the onion and jalapeño in the avocado oil over medium-high heat until they begin to soften. Add the mushrooms and stir constantly until everything softens further. Remove the pan from the heat.

5. Scoop the sweet potato flesh from their skins (reserve the skins), mash, and mix with the vegetable mixture.
6. Add the cumin, paprika, salt and pepper to the mixture.
7. Stuff the mixture back into the potato skins. Bake another 15 minutes if desired. Sprinkle with parsley, if desired.

*Per serving (½ whole sweet potato): 70 calories, 1g fat, 0g saturated fat, 0mg cholesterol, 40mg sodium, 15g carbohydrates, 2g fiber, 2g protein*

## LEMON ARTICHOKES

Yields: 6 servings

### Ingredients

2 (14-ounce) bags frozen artichoke bottoms, defrosted and quartered
½ cup fresh lemon juice
¼ cup extra-virgin olive oil
1 tsp. garlic powder
1 tsp. salt

### Directions

1. Preheat the oven to 350°F.
2. Place the artichokes in a 9x13-inch oven-proof baking dish. Combine the lemon juice, olive oil, salt, and garlic powder, and spread over the artichokes.
3. Bake, covered, for 1½ hours, or until very soft; uncover and bake for 20 minutes longer.

*Per serving: 120 calories, 9g fat, 1.5 saturated fat, 0mg cholesterol, 40mg sodium, 8g carbohydrates, 3g fiber, 2g protein*

# DAY TEN

## Mindful Meditation to Start Your Day

*"Gam Ze Ya'avor."*
*(This too shall pass.)*
—JEWISH FOLKLORE

There's a story about King Solomon, who once asked someone to find him something to wear that, "If a happy man looks at it, he becomes sad, and if a sad man looks at it, he becomes happy." His most trusted servant searched far and wide and found a ring with the transcription, "Gam Ze Ya'avor." The statement evokes an eternal truth that whatever you are going through or may be feeling, whether happy or sad, is transient—it can change in an instant.

On Day 10, you are midway through your 21-day kosher girl's diet. It's natural that overwhelming feelings pop up as you look at the road ahead. However, do not become a victim to negative thoughts and think you have to accept them. As intense as the emotions may be now, they will quickly pass. Remind yourself of why you embarked on the journey of the diet. Look at how far you have come and think about all you accomplished thus far. Stay positive and focused; you are halfway there!

## For Starters

 **Kosher Cleanse Elixir:** Drink upon waking (see page 97).

 **Daily Fitness Goal:** Ease back with muscle recovery by resting today, or perform a yoga stretch of your choice. Don't forget to walk your 10,000 steps today!

## Breakfast

• **Overnight Oats**

## Snack

• ¾ **RX Bar**

## Lunch

• 4 ounces **Grilled Tuna** on a large salad filled with non-starchy veggies and 2 tbsp. any choice of dressing with ½ cup **Butternut Squash Soup**

## Snack

• ¼ avocado with 1 or more bell peppers

## Dinner

• 4 ounces **Turkey Burger** with 1 tbsp. of raw sauerkraut and ½ cup **In a Jiffy Bean Salad**

---

 **BETH'S PREP TIPS**

Prep the air-popped popcorn for tomorrow's snack if you don't have time to make it tomorrow.

# Day Ten Recipes

## OVERNIGHT OATS

Yield: 1 serving

### Ingredients

⅓ cup rolled oats
⅓ to ½ cup unsweetened almond milk
⅓ cup plain Greek yogurt
½ banana or 1/3 cup other fresh fruit
1 tbsp. chia seeds
Pinch ground cinnamon

### Directions

Stir the oats, almond milk, Greek yogurt, fruit, chia seeds, and cinnamon together in a bowl until combined. Transfer to a jar and refrigerate overnight.

*Per serving: 265 calories, 6g fat, 1g saturated fat, 114mg sodium, 3mg cholesterol, 41g carbohydrates, 10g fiber, 14g protein*

## GRILLED TUNA SEASONING

You can season both sides of the tuna with Montreal Steak Seasoning or create your own spice combination for a cleaner version.

### Ingredients

2 tbsp. paprika
2 tbsp. black pepper
2 tbsp. Kosher salt
1 tbsp. garlic powder
1 tbsp. granulated onion
1 tbsp. crushed coriander
1 tbsp. dried dill
1 tbsp. crushed red pepper flakes

### Directions

Mix ingredients together and store in an airtight container.

(Source: chowhound.com)

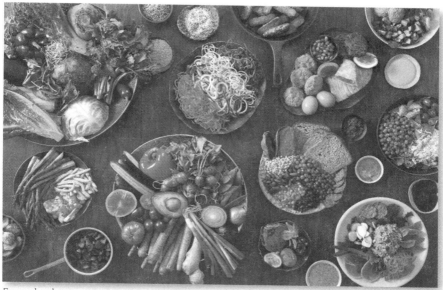

For a color photo, see page 184-185.

## TURKEY BURGER

Yield: 1 serving

### Ingredients

4 ounces lean ground turkey breast
½ garlic clove, minced
2 tsp. finely chopped fresh parsley
½ tsp. finely chopped fresh rosemary
Nonstick cooking spray

### Directions

1. Using your hands, mix the turkey, garlic, parsley, and rosemary until well combined. Flatten into a patty.
2. Heat a small skillet and spray with nonstick cooking spray. Cook the turkey patty 6 minutes on each side. You can always pile on more veggies to your burger such as tomatoes, onions, and peppers, for example.

*Per serving: 120 calories, 2g fat, 0g saturated fat, 50mg cholesterol, 80mg sodium, 6g carbo-hydrates, 1g fiber, 20g protein*

# DAY ELEVEN

## Mindful Meditation to Start Your Day

*"No disease that can be treated by diet should be
treated with any other means."*

—MAIMONIDES, MEDICAL APHORISMS OF MOSES MAIMONIDES

Remember those benefits outside of weight loss that you're experiencing while on my kosher girl's diet? By Day 11, you are fully engaged in altering your entire internal processes and heading towards achieving the goal of improving your state of health through diet. The kosher whole foods you are eating promote an anti-inflammatory state within your body. Chronic inflammation, which is promoted by eating heavily processed foods, is connected to most diseases including cancer, Alzheimer's, and cardiovascular disease. Plus, my diet advocates fitness, which not only helps with weight, but is also an independent positive factor in improving your health. By taking the steps to lose weight, you are taking leaps for your health by being on this diet. With the combined impact of transforming your overall state of physical and emotional health, you are setting the foundation for the weight loss results that last.

# For Starters

 **Kosher Cleanse Elixir:** Drink upon waking (see page 97).

 **Daily Fitness Goal:** Speaking of targeting fat loss, focus on those areas everyone likes to work in this "HIIT workout for abs and obliques" (youtu.be/hyFIKDLmYyo) and walk, walk, walk!

# Breakfast

- **3 Ingredient Pancake**

# Snack

- Trail Mix 100 calories (½ ounce raw nuts and 1 tbsp. raisins or dried cranberries)

# Lunch

- **Asian Tempeh Salad**

# Snack

- 1 cup air-popped popcorn with 1 tsp. nutritional yeast

# Dinner

- 1 cup unsweetened fennel tea, hot or iced 🍵
- 4 ounces **Miso Glazed Salmon** with **Cauliflower "Rice"** and roasted broccoli

## 🍽️ BETH'S PREP TIPS

- ¼ cup organic popcorn kernels makes about 4 cups of popped corn.
- You can purchase a store-bought unsalted trail mix that is 100 calories containing only raw nuts and dried fruit with no added sugar.
- Refrigerate extra tempeh to eat at lunch on Day 19.

# Day Eleven Recipes

## 3 INGREDIENT PANCAKE

Yield: 1 serving

### Ingredients

½ banana
1 egg
⅛ tsp. baking powder
Pinch of ground cinnamon
Nonstick cooking spray

### Directions

1. Mash the banana in a bowl using a fork; add the egg, baking powder, and cinnamon, and mix the batter well.
2. Spritz nonstick cooking spray in a skillet over medium heat. Spoon batter into the skillet and cook until bubbles form and the edges are dry, 2 to 3 minutes. Flip and cook until browned on the other side, 2 to 3 minutes.

*Per serving: 120 calories, 5g fat, 1.5g saturated fat, 185mg cholesterol, 70 mg sodium, 14g carbohydrates, 2g fiber, 7g protein*

## ASIAN TEMPEH SALAD

### Ingredients

2 to 3 cups kale
2 tsp. extra-virgin olive oil
4 **Marinated Tempeh** slices
½ cup farro, cooked according to package directions
1 handful purple cabbage, shredded
2 tbsp. tuxedo sesame seeds
2 tbsp. **Miso Dressing**

### Directions

1. Preheat the oven to 350°F.
2. Bake the tempeh for 18 minutes, flipping halfway at the 9-minute mark.
3. Combine the kale and olive oil. Massage the kale to soften the ribs with your hands.
4. Arrange the salad with the kale, tempeh, farro, and cabbage, and top with the sesame seeds and dressing.

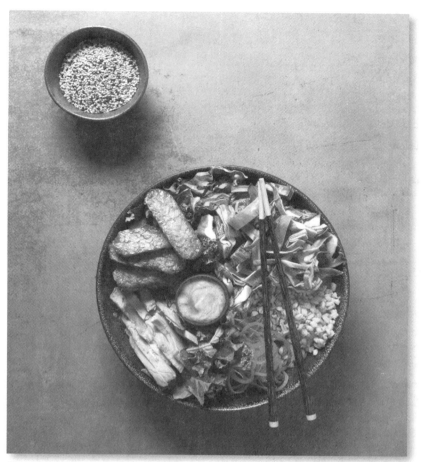

*For a color photo, see page 187.*

## MARINATED TEMPEH

### Ingredients

⅛ cup soy sauce
2 tbsp. raw honey, melted
1 (8-ounce) package of tempeh, sliced

### Directions

Combine the soy sauce and honey. Marinate the tempeh at least 30 minutes in honey and soy sauce.

## MISO GLAZED SALMON

Yield: 1 serving

### Ingredients

1½ tbsp. white miso
1 tsp. agave syrup
½ tsp. avocado oil
4 to 6 ounces wild salmon fillets

### Directions

1.  Set the oven to Broil.
2.  In a small bowl mix the miso, agave syrup, and avocado oil.
3.  Spread the marinade over the salmon and broil until cooked through, about 8 to 10 minutes.

*Per serving: 210 calories, 8g fat, 1g saturated fat, 60mg cholesterol, 51g sodium 6.5g carbo-hydrates, 1g fiber, 25g protein*

## CAULIFLOWER "RICE"

Yield: 1 serving

### Ingredients

1 head cauliflower, separated into florets
1 tbsp. extra-virgin olive oil
Salt and pepper, to taste

### Directions

1.  Place the cauliflower into in a food processor and process 1 to 2 minutes or until a "rice-like" consistency is reached.
2.  Heat the olive oil in a skillet over medium heat; add the cauliflower "rice," and the salt and pepper. Cover the skillet and cook until heated through (3 to 5 minutes).
3.  Remove lid and fluff the "rice" with a fork.

*Per serving: 187 calories, 13.5g fat, 1g saturated fat, 0mg cholesterol, 155mg sodium, 14g carbo-hydrates, 7g fiber, 5g protein*

# DAY TWELVE

# SABBATH NIGHT

## Mindful Meditation to Start Your Day

*"Who acts from love is greater than who acts from fear."*
—TALMUD, SOTA 31A

A concept in the Talmud discusses the impact of doing something in a state of love versus a state of fear. With my experience counseling clients and witnessing in the way I talk to myself, I see firsthand the lasting impacts of change from a place of love and positivity. Oftentimes, I hear people talk about themselves negatively, or they rely on people for weight loss advice who invoke fear of foods and imperfection. A diet cannot be maintained long-term from heavy restrictions, negative self-talk, and fear of failure. Success on a diet is not about perfection; it is about making yourself do better and continuously improve each day. It's about "rolling with the punches" of the inevitable unknowns of everyday living and picking yourself back up even stronger and more driven.

By allowing your mindset to embrace degrees of flexibility, you will take pressure off your shoulders that strives for perfection. You are living in an imperfect world with unexpected obstacles in your path. If you don't keep your thoughts positive and shrug off negative scenarios, you will fall out from your weight loss goals. For example, you'll eat a salad at each meal, but sometimes you grab some Persian cucumbers when you are rushed, and that's okay. If you are too rigid in your expectations, then you won't see there is always a way to make it work.

## For Starters

 **Kosher Cleanse Elixir:** Drink upon waking (see page 97).

 **Daily Fitness Goal:** Try targeting your full body today with this 30-Minute Fat-Burning Cardio Sculpt Workout (youtube.com/watch?v=QsiImYTLvTk), plus get your walking in!

## Breakfast

- **Flavorful Omelet** with 1 cup cubed honeydew

## Snack

- 1 **Kind Bar** with less than 5g sugar

## Lunch

- 1 cup shelled edamame combined with a large salad filled with nonstarchy veggies, ½ cup organic corn niblets, and ¼ avocado with 2 tbsp. of **Miso Dressing**

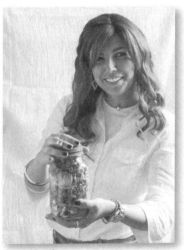

## Snack

- ½ cup cottage cheese sprinkled with ground cinnamon and 1 cup of cubed cantaloupe

*For a color photo, see page 188.*

## Dinner

- 1 cup unsweetened mint tea, hot or iced
- 4 ounces red wine (counts as an after-dinner optional snack) if this is your Sabbath night meal
- 3 ounces **Grass-fed Pepper Steak**
- ½ cup cooked **Wild Rice with Almonds and Cherries** (or substitute the "challah" whole wheat sourdough bread instead of the wild rice)

 **BETH'S PREP TIPS**

Prepare the **Roasted Chickpeas** for tomorrow's dinner and the Grilled Chicken for tomorrow's lunch!

# Day Twelve Recipes

## FLAVORFUL OMELET

Yield: 1 serving

### Ingredients

3 egg whites and one egg yolk
1 tbsp. unsweetened almond milk
1 tsp. extra-virgin olive oil
¼ tsp. brown mustard seeds
⅛ tsp. turmeric
2 green onions, finely chopped, white and light green parts only
¼ cup diced plum tomato
¼ cup diced bell pepper
Handful diced baby spinach leaves (optional)
Salt, to taste
Fresh black pepper, to taste

### Directions

1. Whisk together the eggs, milk, salt, and pepper. Set aside.
2. Heat the olive oil in a large skillet (ideally cast-iron) over medium-high heat. Add the scallions, mustard seeds and turmeric.
3. Cook 30 seconds or until the scallions soften, stirring often.
4. Add the tomato and peppers and cook about 1 minute, stirring frequently.
5. Pour the egg mixture into the pan. Spread the mixture around so that it spreads evenly.
6. Cook about 2 minutes until the edges of the egg mixture start to brown; flip to cook the other side.

*Per serving: 180 calories, 8g fat, 1.5g saturated fat, 65mg cholesterol, 180mg sodium, 16g carbo-hydrates, 4g fiber, 13g protein*

## GRASS-FED PEPPER STEAK

Yield: 8 servings

### Ingredients

6 tsp. taco seasoning (see the following recipe)
2½ lbs. grass-fed beefsteak
1 tbsp. extra-virgin olive oil
1 onion, chopped
1 package baby peppers

*(recipe continues, page 160)*

### Directions

1. Rub the taco seasoning on the meat.
2. In a skillet over medium heat, brown the meat in the olive oil.
3. Remove the meat from the pan, but leave its juices.
4. Add the onion and peppers to the skillet and sauté until soft.
5. Add the meat and cook on low for 5 minutes.

*Per serving (3 ounces): 320 calories, 19g fat, 7g saturated fat, 85mg cholesterol, 690 mg sodium, 6g carbohydrates, 1g fiber, 27g protein*

## TACO SEASONING

### Ingredients

6 tsp. chili powder
5 tsp. paprika
4½ tsp. ground cumin
3 tsp. onion powder
2½ tsp. garlic powder
⅛ tsp. cayenne pepper

### Directions

Combine all the ingredients and mix well. Store in airtight container.

## WILD RICE WITH ALMONDS AND CHERRIES

Yield: 6 servings

### Ingredients

1 onion, chopped
1 tbsp. extra-virgin olive oil
1 cup wild rice
2 cups low-sodium organic vegetable broth
¼ cup sliced almonds
1/8 cup dried cherries (no sugar added), cut the cherries into pieces
Salt and pepper, to taste

### Directions

1. In a medium saucepan, sauté the onion in olive oil until softened.
2. Add the wild rice and broth.
3. Season with salt and pepper, lower the heat, and cover.
4. Cook about 20 more minutes.
5. Add the almonds and cherries, and salt and pepper to taste.

*Per serving: 160 calories, 4.5g fat, 0.5g saturated fat, 320 sodium, 0mg cholesterol, 26g carbohydrates, 3g fiber, 5g protein*

# DAY THIRTEEN

## SABBATH DAY

## Mindful Meditation to Start Your Day

*"Though the righteous one may fall seven times,*
*he will arise."*

—PROVERBS 24:16

In Jewish thinking, a great person isn't one who never fails; it's one who fails and keeps trying. You can only become a truly great person through the crucible of failure and perseverance.*

Sometimes life experiences feel as if they are burying you alive and ifficult situations make you feel like there is no way out. When it comes to your diet and health, there is always a way to break out of the defeating feeling of failed weight loss effort. You have a tremendous ability to change your palate and workings of your digestive system. If you put effort in the areas that are proven effective, you will see changes occur over time. It may seem as if it is a slow journey, but at the end of the 21 days on my diet you will look back in awe of your transformation.

In other single-minded fad diets, you are asked to do part of the work. For example, simply calorie counting or only exercising to lose weight may accomplish some degree of weight loss, yet because of the minimal effort in only one area the results are short-lived. By making changes in only one aspect involved in weight loss, you are not digging

---

* aish.com/sp/pg/Inspiring-Jewish-Quotes-for-Rosh-Hashanah.html

deep into what will effectively change your habits in order to maintain the weight loss, nor will you experience other benefits to your overall health. It takes picking yourself back up and perform a true lifestyle and diet overhaul to make the hard-earned results last. As this quote from the Talmud infers, you may feel you keep failing in your weight loss efforts, but you will persevere if you keep on pushing towards your goal with the right plan. You can do this, keep it up!

## For Starters

 **Kosher Cleanse Elixir:** Drink upon waking (see page 97).

 **Daily Fitness Goal:** Aside from walking, take your weekly Sabbath rest.

## Breakfast

- 6 ounces plain Greek yogurt with 1 cup mixed berries and 1 tsp. chia seeds

## Snack

- ¼ avocado with 1 or more Persian cucumbers

## Lunch

- 2 ounces whole wheat sourdough bread (if "challah" is mandatory, otherwise eat the beets in the salad)
- 4 ounces grilled chicken breast with **Sesame Mustard String Beans** and choice of large salad with ½ cup of beets (if not eating sourdough bread)

## Snack

- 3 **Almond Date Balls**

## Dinner

- 4 ounces individual tuna on a large salad filled with non-starchy veggies plus **Roasted Moroccan Chickpeas** with 2 tbsp. **Miso Dressing**

**BETH'S PREP TIPS**

- If you don't have time or forget to prepare the fresh chickpeas, you can use canned chickpeas. Simply rinse and rub off the outer layer on each chickpea, then pat dry.
- Roasted Chickpeas are used again on Days 14 and 20 (½ cup serving each). Store in a brown paper bag at room temperature.

# Day Thirteen Recipes

## SESAME MUSTARD STRING BEANS

Yields: 2 servings

### Ingredients

1 lb. string beans, frozen or fresh
2 tbsp. Dijon mustard
1 tsp. extra-virgin olive oil
1 tbsp. sesame seeds

### Directions

1. Preheat the oven to 425°F.
2. Spread the string beans on a baking sheet lined with parchment paper.
3. Combine the mustard, olive oil, and sesame seeds into a bowl and brush onto the string beans.
4. Roast for 20 minutes or until desired crispness.

*Per serving: 188 calories, 9g fat, 1g saturated fat, 301mg sodium, 0mg cholesterol, 21g carbohydrate, 8g fiber, 4g protein*

## ROASTED MOROCCAN CHICKPEAS

Yields: 4 servings

### Ingredients

8 ounces fresh chickpeas, soaked overnight
1 tbsp. extra-virgin olive oil
½ tsp. ground cumin
¼ tsp. cayenne
¼ tsp. ground cinnamon
¼ tsp. garlic powder
¼ tsp. paprika
¼ tsp. Kosher salt

*(recipe continues, page 164)*

## Directions

1. Soak chickpeas overnight or at least 8 hours in the refrigerator. The water should cover the chickpeas completely.
2. Preheat the oven to 400°F.
3. Line a baking sheet with parchment paper. Rinse the chickpeas well and pat them dry between two paper towels. Place on the baking sheet. Drizzle the chickpeas with the olive oil and roast in the middle rack of the oven, tossing every 15 minutes, until deep golden, dry, and crunchy, about 40 to 45 minutes.
4. While the chickpeas roast, combine the cumin, cayenne, cinnamon, garlic powder, paprika, and salt in a medium bowl. Mix until the color is uniform.
5. As soon as the chickpeas come out of the oven, toss with the spice blend.

*Per serving: 160 calories, 5g fat, .5g saturated, 0g cholesterol, 460mg sodium, 25g carbohydrates, 5g fiber, 5g protein*

# DAY FOURTEEN

## Mindful Meditation to Start Your Day

*"Who guards his mouth and tongue guards himself from troubles."*

—PROVERBS 21:23

We can interpret "mouth" as a reference to protecting yourself from excessive and unhealthy food and "tongue" from inappropriate speech. The added effort to protect your mouth and tongue against unhealthy foods and talk will ultimately prevent you from getting into trouble for your emotional and physical health. Throughout the 21 days, your guard is up against tempting foods off the diet plan. There is a large element of thought following you throughout the day to ensure you are staying on track and thinking of the next meal or snack so that you are prepared. Although overwhelming at times, the thought involved in preparation and planning is key in keeping you focused on the plan and lessen the temptation to grab at something less healthy around you. By revolving your thoughts, not only your mouth, around the plan each day, you are leaving no room for error in getting results on the diet. In other words, it may feel as if you are thinking about food all day, but the thoughtfulness is worth the resulting success.

## For Starters

 **Kosher Cleanse Elixir:** Drink upon waking (see page 97).

 **Daily Fitness Goal:** Ease into the diet with a boost of motivation and physical fitness from your choice of yoga routine for 15 minutes (see examples). Don't forget to walk your 10,000 steps today!

## Breakfast

- Omelet consisting of 3 egg whites and 1 egg yolk, seasoned with your choice of spices, such as zaatar spice, plus 1 peach

## Snack

- 1 tbsp. almond butter with 1 or more celery stalks

## Lunch

- 2 **Gal's Black Bean Burgers**
- A large salad filled with non-starchy veggies and 2 tbsp. of any choice of dressing with ½ roasted sweet potato

## Snack

- ½ cup **Roasted Chickpeas**

## Dinner

- **Quinoa Crust Pizza** with loads of non-starchy veggies piled on top or on the side

 **BETH'S PREP TIPS**

- Simply pop your frozen veggie burgers you made in advance into the toaster; however, the recipe is referenced again in the event you need to make more.
- Use ½ cup of the stored Roasted Chickpeas. Keep another ½ cup reserved because Roasted Chickpeas are used again on Day 20.

# Day Fourteen Recipes

## GAL'S BLACK BEAN BURGERS

Yield: 6 servings

### Ingredients

¼ white onion, grated
1 (15-ounce) can black beans rinsed, drained, and mashed
½ cup oat flour (¾ cup oats ground into flour)
⅓ cup parsley, chopped
1 tbsp. tomato paste
1½ tbsp. Cajun seasoning
1 tbsp. ground flaxseed
Salt and pepper, to taste

### Directions

1. Preheat the oven to 350°F.
2. Combine all ingredients in a large bowl.
3. Form into 6 regular-sized burgers.
4. Bake about 8 minutes on each side.

*Per serving: 100 calories, 1.5g fat, 0g saturated fat, 0mg cholesterol, 850mg sodium, 17g carbs, 5g fiber, 5g protein*

## QUINOA CRUST PIZZA

Yield: 1 serving

### Ingredients

¾ cup uncooked quinoa
¼ cup water
1 tsp. baking powder
¼ tsp. salt
1 ounce mozzarella cheese
2 tbsp. tomato sauce
Choice of toppings, such as fresh arugula
   and sundried tomatoes

### Directions

1. Place uncooked quinoa in a small bowl and cover with water. Let the quinoa soak overnight or for at least 8 hours.
2. Preheat the oven to 425°F.

*(recipe continues, page 168)*

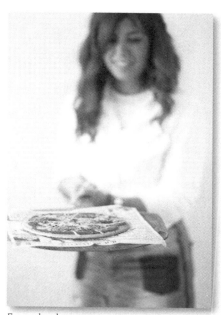

*For a color photo, see page 189.*

3. Drain and thoroughly rinse the quinoa to prevent any bitterness in the crust. Place the quinoa, water, baking powder, and salt in the bowl of a food processor. Process until a smooth batter is formed, about 2 minutes, scraping down the sides of the food processor as necessary.
4. Line an 8- or 9-inch round cake pan with parchment paper (it may help to spray the pan with cooking spray first, so that the parchment sticks), and then spray the parchment paper with cooking spray. Pour the batter into the pan and smooth with a rubber spatula.
5. Bake the crust for 15 minutes, and flip out of the cake pan. Remove the parchment paper from the crust.
6. Flip the crust over and return to the oven for 5 to 10 more minutes, or until golden and the edges are crispy.
7. Remove from the oven and add the cheese, sauce, and toppings of your choice.
8. Return to the oven and bake another 10 minutes, or until the cheese is melty.

*Per Serving: 400 calories, 10g fat, 3.5g saturated fat, 20mg cholesterol, 520mg sodium, 58g carbohydrate, 6g fiber, 19g protein*

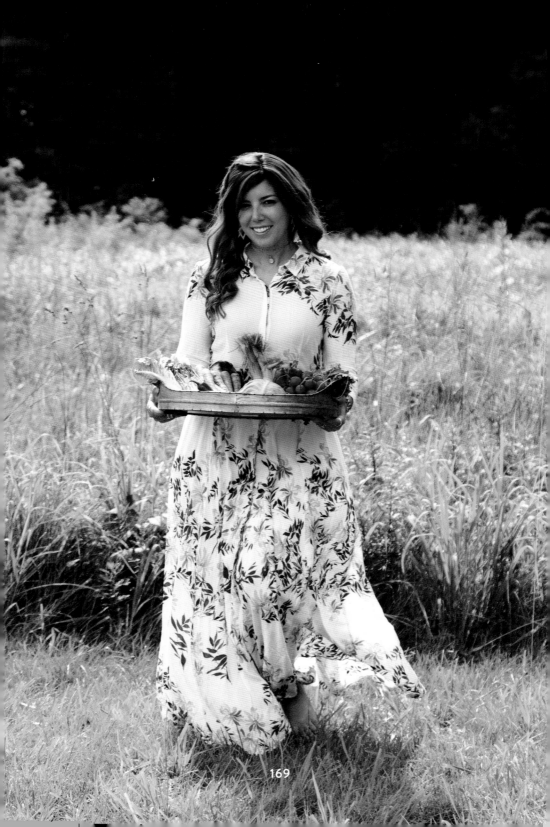

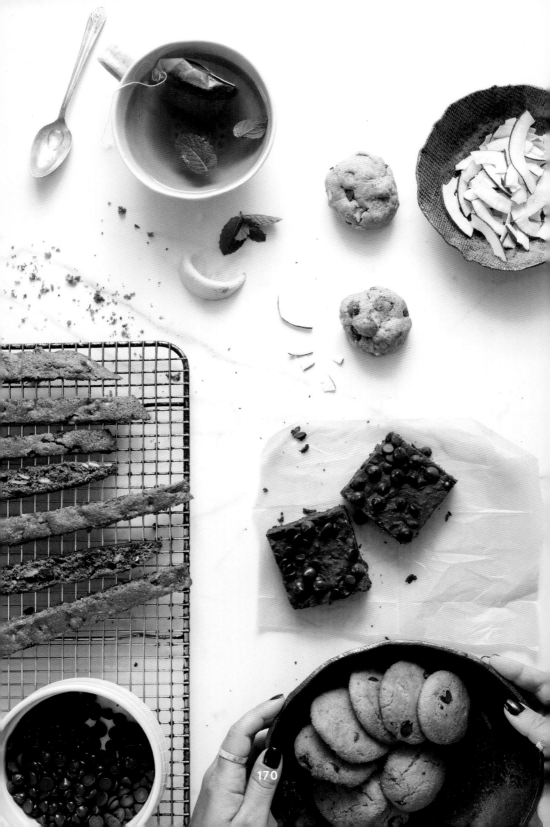

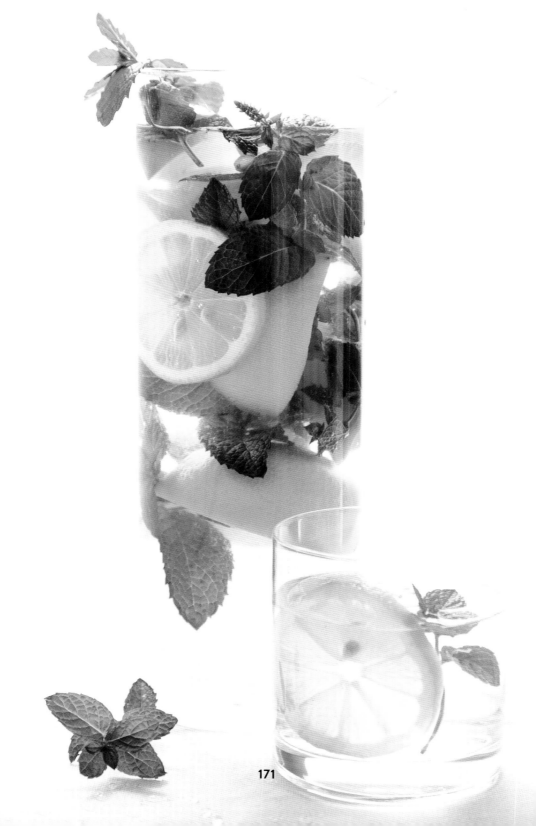

171

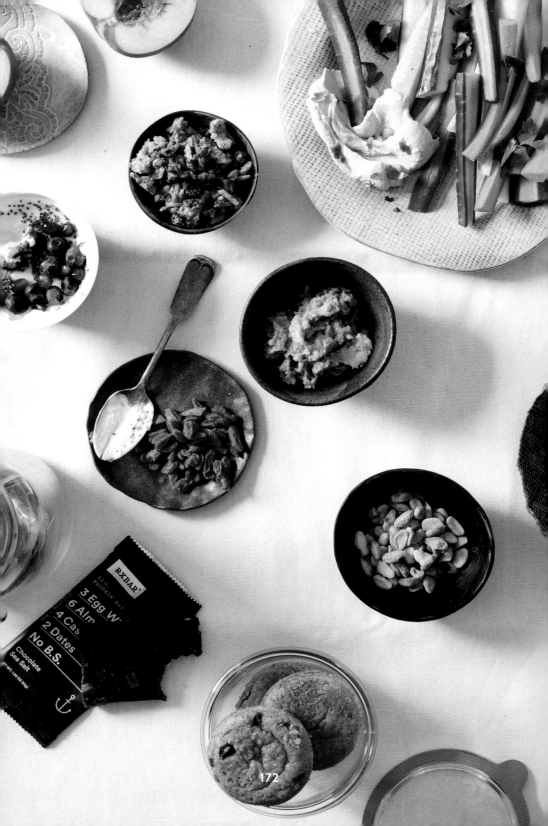

RXBAR
12 g.
PROTEIN BAR

3 Egg Wh
6 Alm
4 Cas
2 Dates
No B.S.

Chocolate
Sea Salt
NET WT. 1.83 OZ (52g)

172

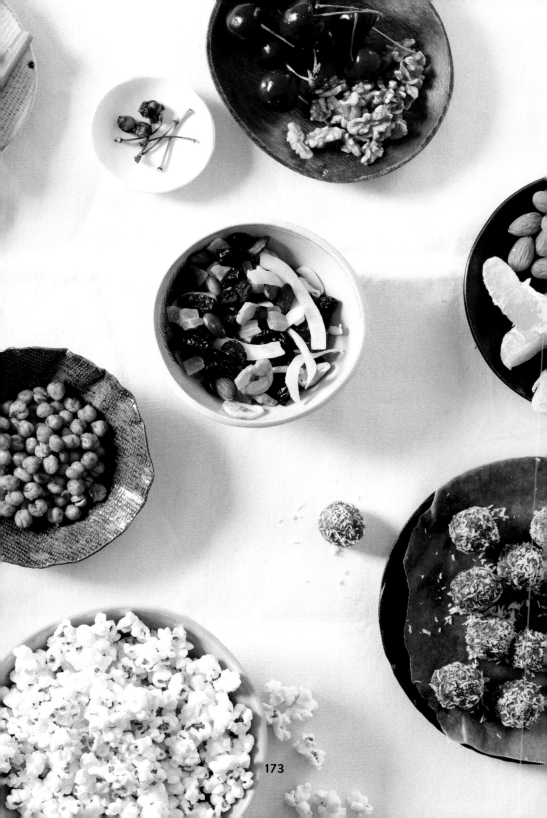

173

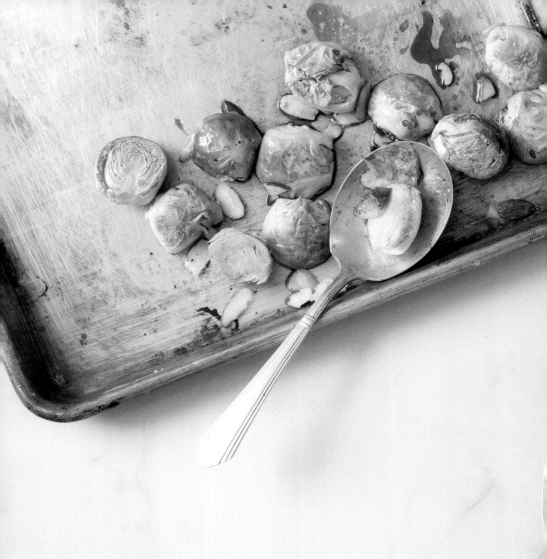

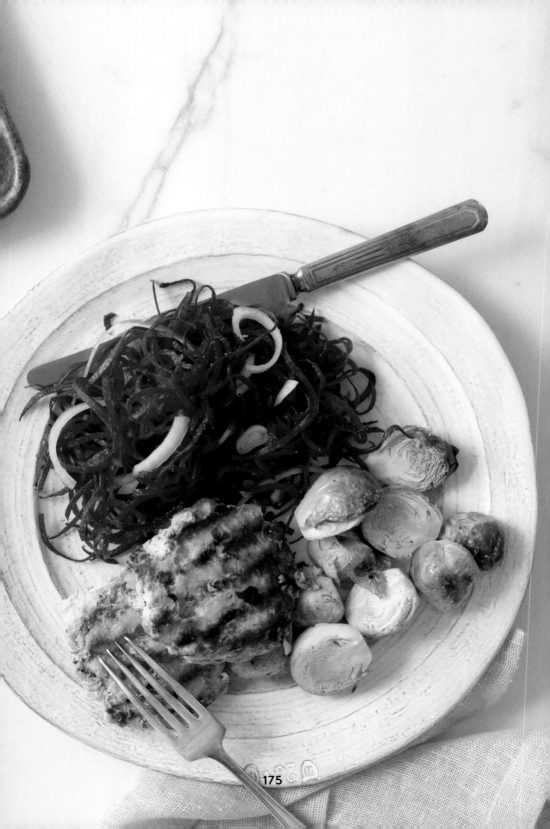

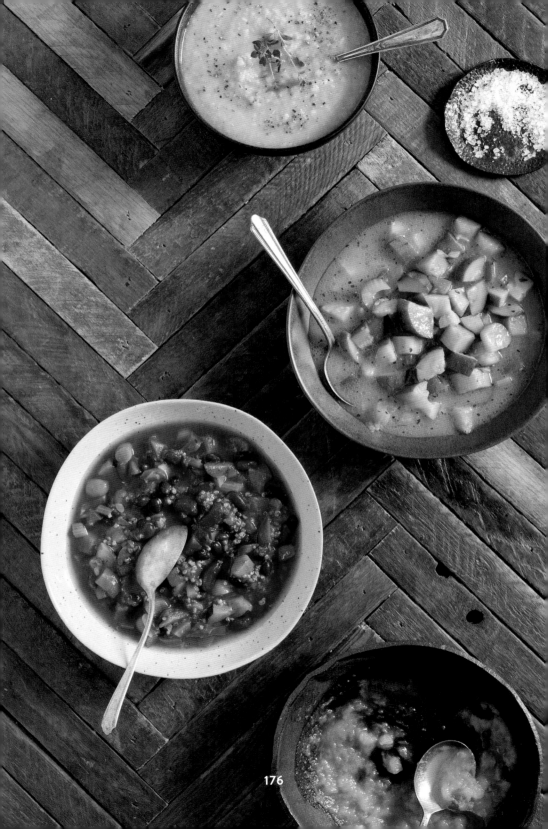

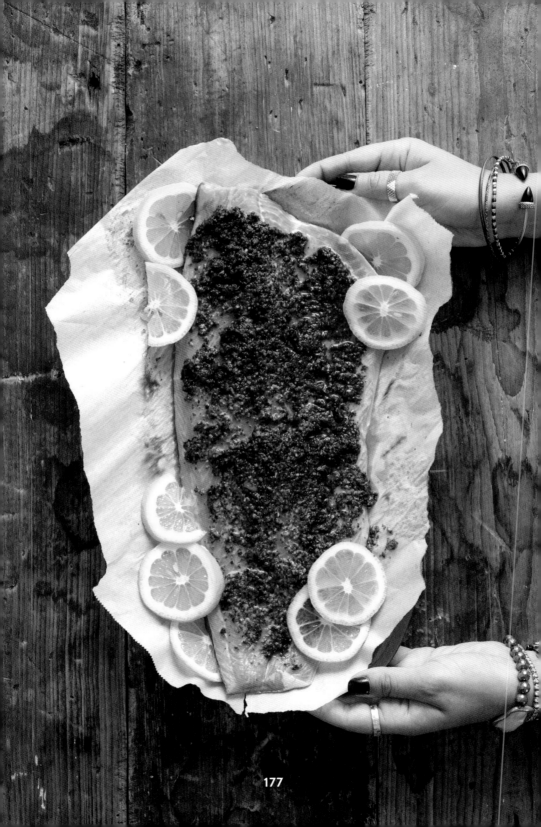

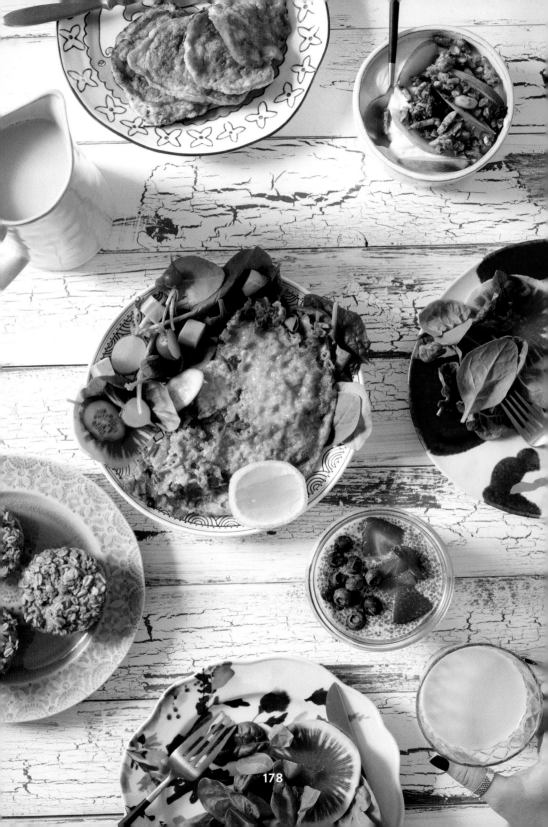

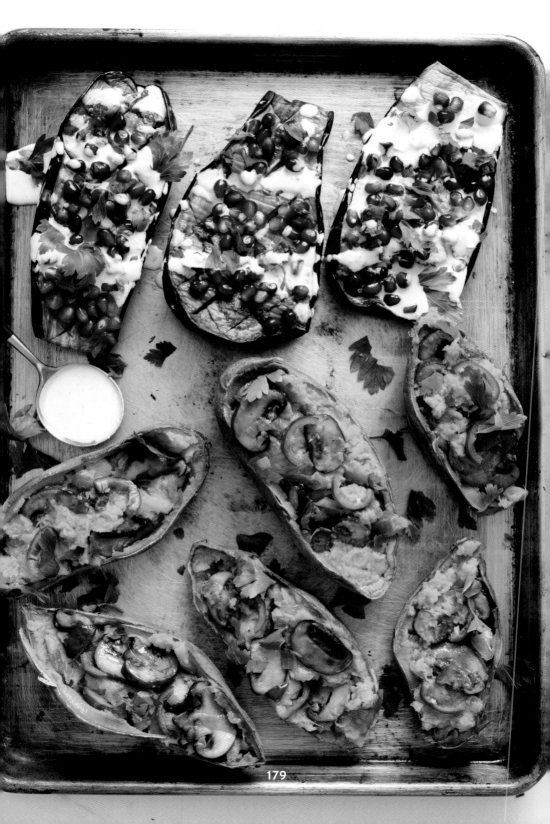

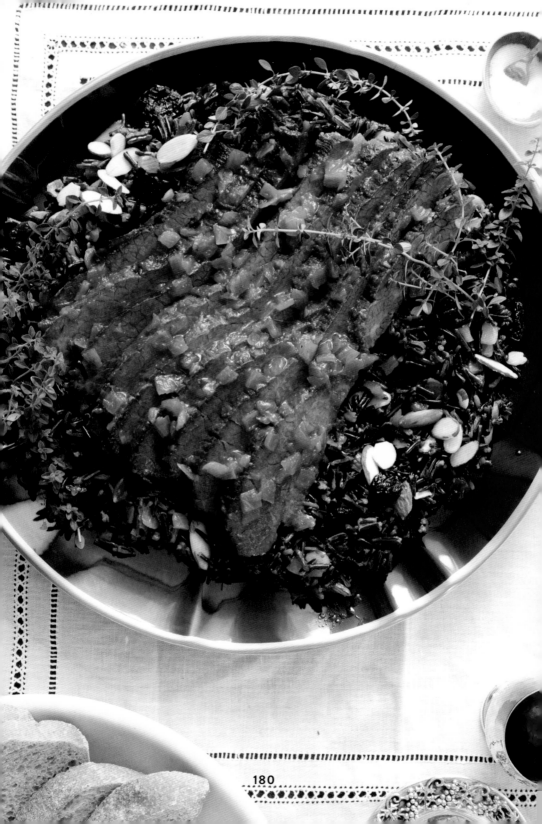

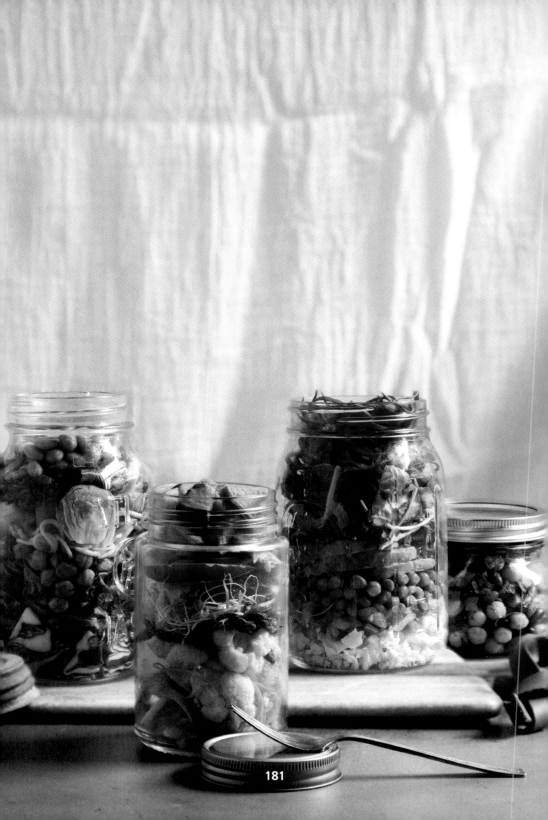

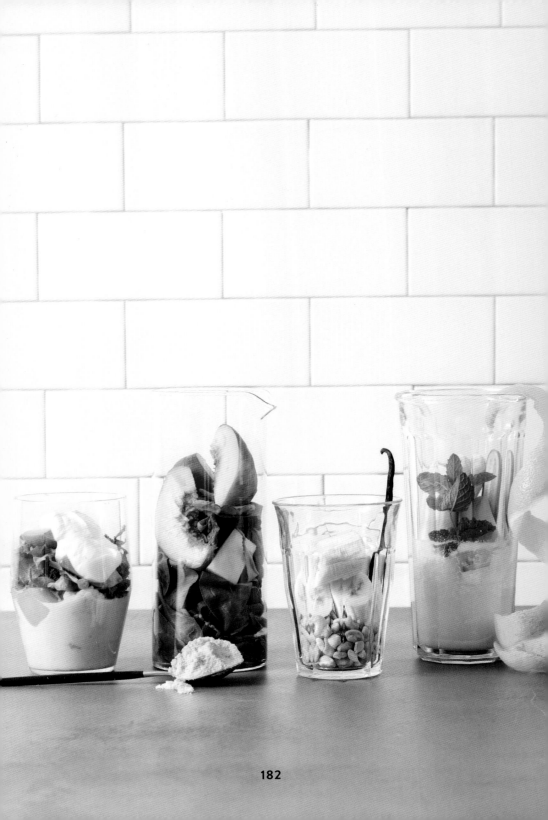

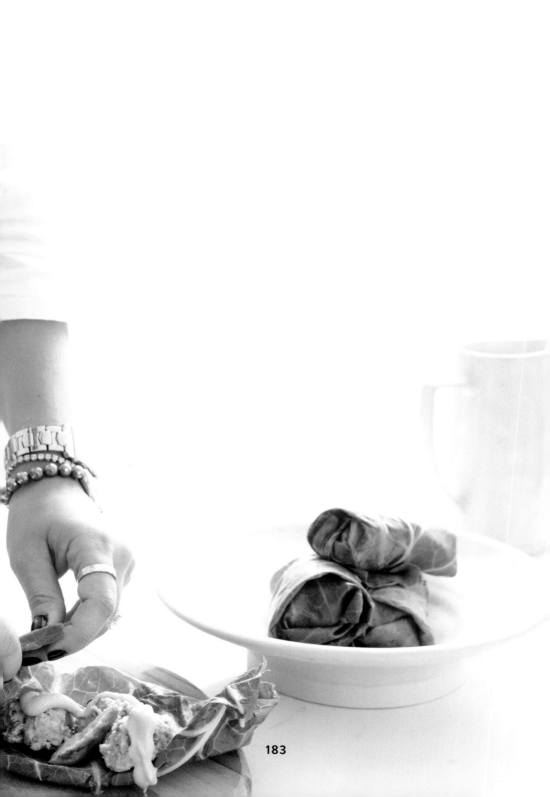

183

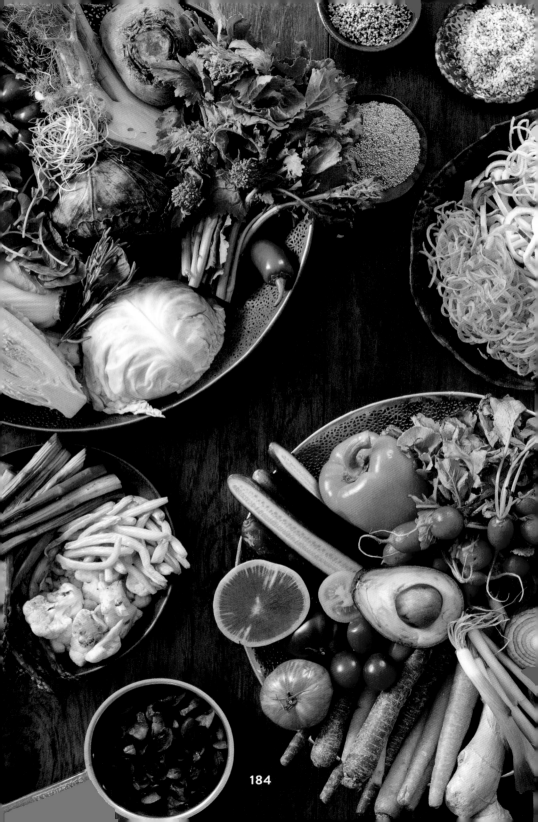

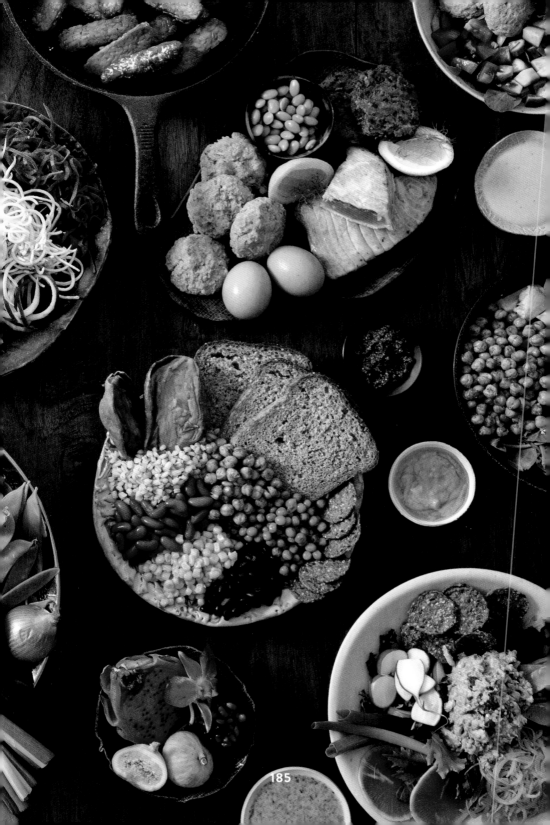

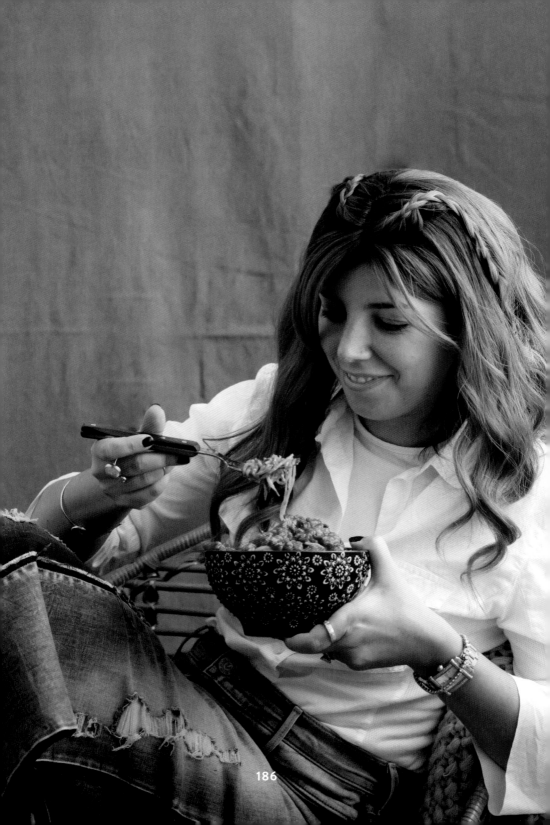

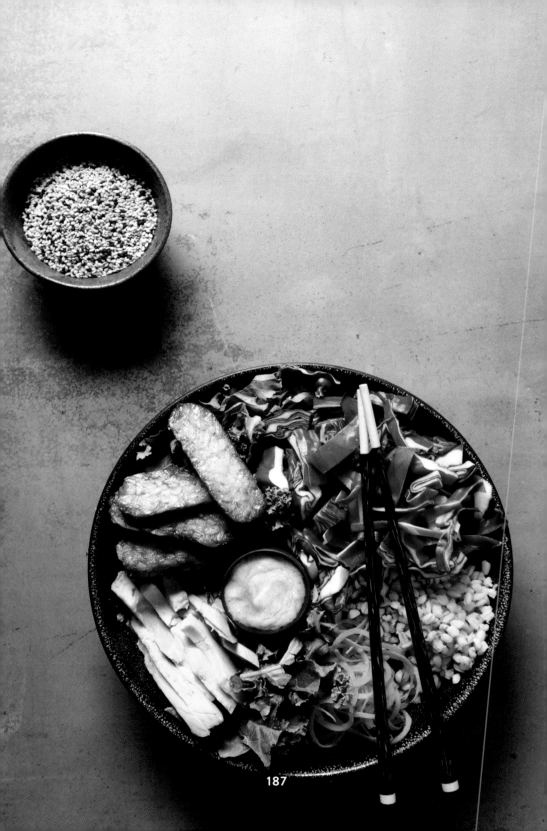

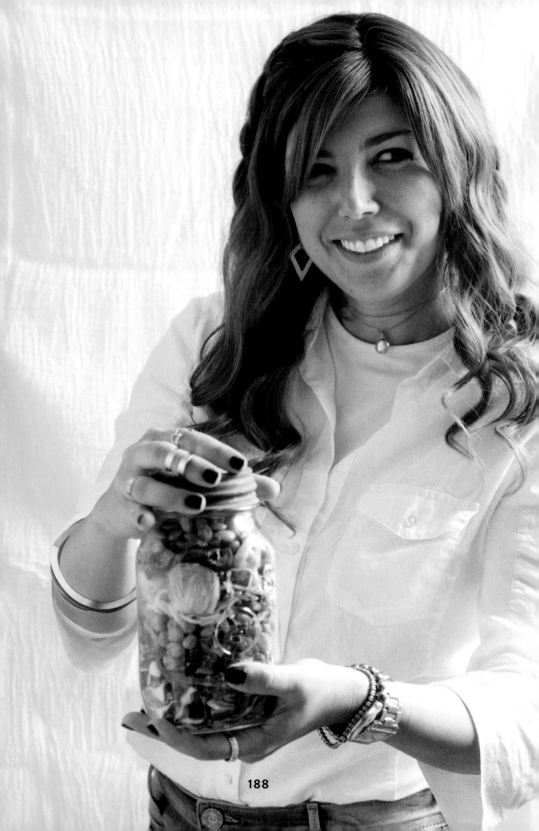

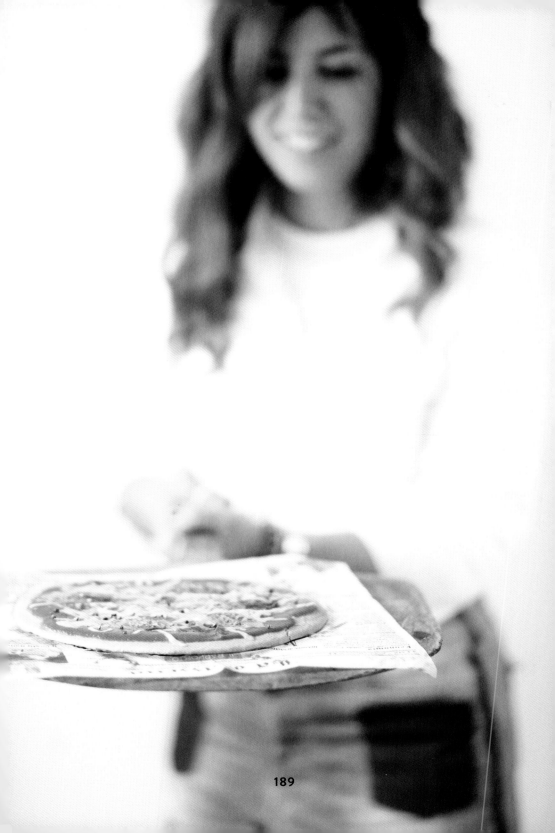

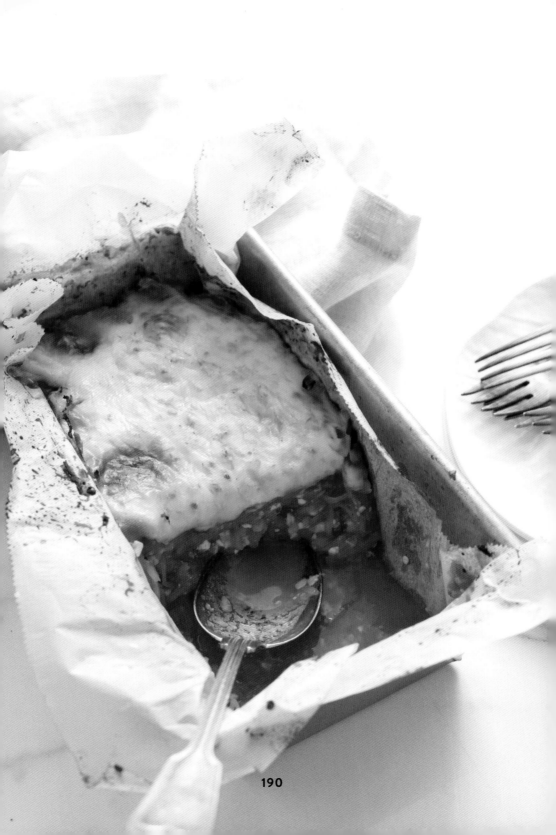

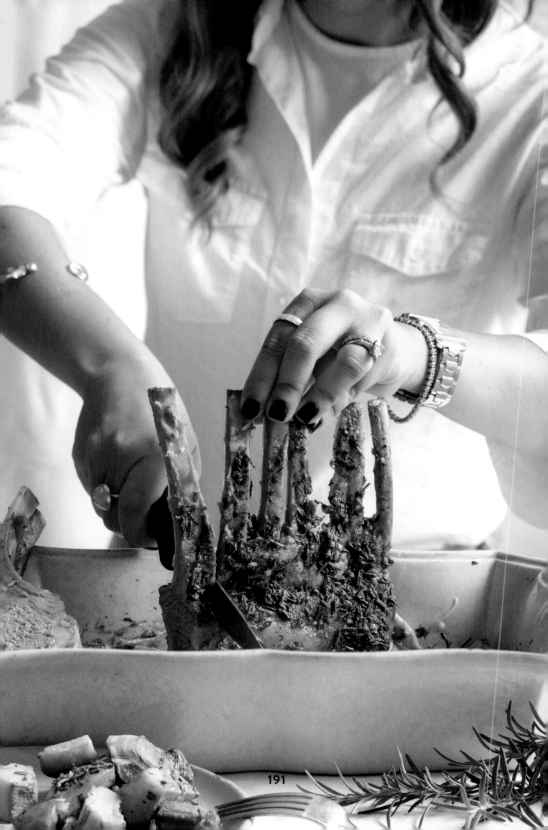

191

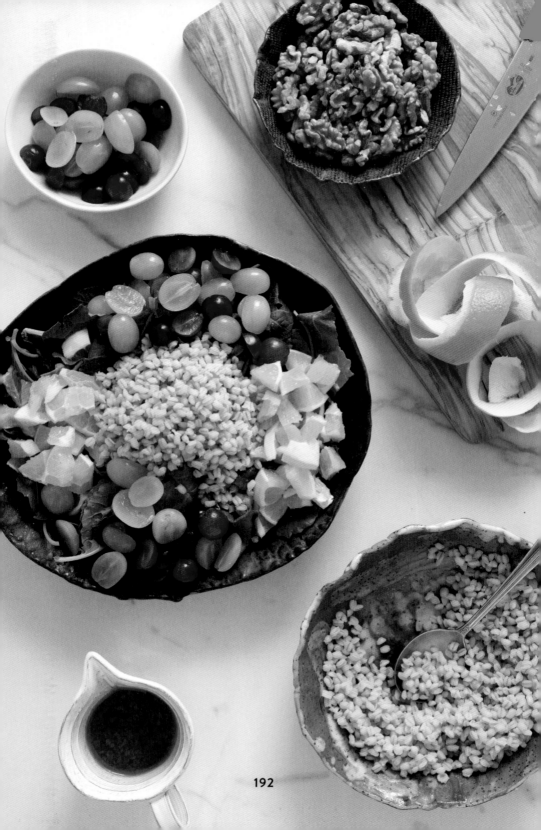

# DAY FIFTEEN

## Mindful Meditation to Start Your Day

*"If you believe breaking is possible,*
*believe fixing is possible."*

—RABBI NAHMAN OF BRESLOV (1772–1810),
FOUNDER OF THE BRESLOV HASIDIC MOVEMENT

There is always a way to come back from a weak point and become something more. Nothing is impossible. At this stage, you have to trust you can see the diet through until the end. Ultimately, you are your own most meaningful motivator. At times, you may have outside support or people who remark on your weight loss, but those comments are ephemeral. You will be the last one standing with yourself. Only you can get your body to the end of your health goals. Leave the past diet failures and insecurities behind so you can embrace the new you that you are becoming. Just as broken as you thought you were, start to believe what you may have thought impossible: You are getting fixed.

## For Starters

 **Kosher Cleanse Elixir:** Drink upon waking (see page 97).

 **Daily Fitness Goal**: Aside from walking, take a rest while actively stretching with some yoga if you feel up to the fitness challenge.

## Breakfast

• 2 **Almond Butter Muffins** (see Beth's Prep Tip)

## Snack

• ⅛ cup mixed raw nuts with 3 large, round, no-sugar-added dried mango pieces

## Lunch

• 2 **Baked Falafel with Tahini** and large salad filled with non-starchy veggies

## Snack

• 1 **Health Warrior Chia Bar**

## Dinner

• 4 ounces **Lemon Pepper Flounder** with **Roasted Brussel Sprouts** and ½ cup cooked brown rice

 **BETH'S PREP TIPS**

• Freeze the **Almond Butter Muffins**. One is for a snack on Day 17.
• Prepare the **Kale Chips** for tomorrow and store in a brown paper bag if you didn't prepare previously.

# Day Fifteen Recipes

## ALMOND BUTTER MUFFINS

Yields: 12 servings

### Ingredients

2 cups almond flour (almond meal)
2 tsp. baking powder
1 cup unsweetened almond milk
¾ cup almond butter
¼ cup dark chocolate chips, optional

### Directions

1. Preheat the oven to 350°F.
2. In a mixing bowl, combine the almond flour and baking powder.
3. In a separate bowl, stir the almond milk and almond butter together. While whisking, slowly pour the almond flour mixture into the almond milk mixture until combined.
4. Fold in the chocolate chips, if desired. In a paper-lined muffin tray, put about 2 heaping tbsp. of batter inside each muffin tin.
5. Bake about 10 to 15 minutes.

*Per serving: 210 calories, 18g fat, 1.5g saturated fat, 0mg cholesterol, 25mg sodium, 7g carbohydrates, 4g fiber, 7g protein*

## BAKED FALAFEL WITH TAHINI

Yields: 8 Falafel Balls

### Ingredients

1½ cups fresh chickpeas, soaked, or 1 (15-ounce) BPA-free can of chickpeas, rinsed and drained
½ red onion, chopped
2 large garlic cloves, chopped
4 tbsp. chickpea flour
1 tbsp. ground cumin
1 tbsp. ground coriander
2 tbsp. extra-virgin olive oil
1 tbsp. chia seeds + 3 tbsp. water (for egg substitution)
1 small carrot, chopped small
2 tbsp. dried parsley
Sea salt and black pepper, to taste

*(recipe continues, page 172)*

### Directions

1. Combine chia seeds in a bowl and add 3 tbsp. water. Set aside until it forms a gel.
2. Preheat oven to 350°F and line a baking sheet with parchment paper.
3. Combine the chickpeas, onion, garlic, chickpea flour, cumin, coriander, olive oil, salt and pepper, parsley, and carrot. Pulse in a food processor until the mixture is well combined and smooth.
4. Scoop a little less than ¼ cup of the chickpea mixture and form into a ball. Repeat until 8 balls are formed.
5. Bake about 20 to 30 minutes or until the falafel balls are lightly browned on the bottom and golden on top.
6. Remove from oven and allow to cool and harden. Serve with 2 tbsp. of **Tahini Dressing**.

*Per serving (2 balls): 197 calories, 10g fat, 1g saturated fat, 0mg cholesterol, 162mg sodium, 24g carbohydrates, 6g fiber, 7g protein*

## LEMON PEPPER FLOUNDER

Yield: 4 servings

### Ingredients

2 tbsp. grated lemon rind
1 tbsp. extra-virgin olive oil
1¼ tsp. black peppercorns, crushed
½ tsp. salt
2 garlic cloves, minced
4 (6-ounce) flounder fillets
Cooking spray
Lemon wedges, optional

### Directions

1. Preheat the oven to 425°F.
2. Combine the lemon rind, olive oil, peppercorns, salt, and garlic. Place the fillets in a Pyrex dish coated with cooking spray. Rub the lemon-garlic mixture evenly over the fillets.
3. Bake for 8 minutes or until the fish flakes easily when tested with a fork. Serve with lemon wedges, if desired.

*Per serving: 160 calories, 6g fat, 1g saturated fat, 70mg cholesterol, 155mg sodium, 5g carbohydrate, 20g protein*

(Adapted from shecooksshecleans.net)

## BRUSSELS SPROUTS

Servings: 4

### Ingredients

2 cups Brussels sprouts, halved
¼ cup sliced almonds, toasted
Juice of 1 lemon
1 tsp. onion powder
1 tbsp. extra-virgin olive oil
Salt and pepper, to taste

### Directions

1. Preheat the oven to 425°F.
2. Roast Brussels sprouts for about 35 minutes, turning with a spatula once halfway through the cooking. Place in a mixing bowl.
3. Add the almonds, lemon, onion powder, olive oil, and salt and pepper; stir to combine.

*Per serving: 90 calories, 7g fat, 0.5 saturated fat, 0mg cholesterol, 10mg sodium, 6g carbohydrates, 3g fiber, 3g protein*

# DAY SIXTEEN

## Mindful Meditation to Start Your Day

*"Once an error is learned, it is hard to unlearn."*
—TALMUD, BAVA BATRA 21A

Often, I hear people talk down to themselves about aspects of their personality that they do not like but cannot change. The areas include poor habits, such as the difficulties faced when encountering unhealthy foods placed in front of them, and the lack of self-control. Instead of accepting that it is and may always be a challenge to stop themselves from eating tempting foods and working harder to unlearn it, they succumb to the weakness too easily. Subconsciously, this lack of acceptance of their challenges eats away at their self-esteem.

If your self-worth is low, you won't feel empowered to overcome difficulties. It will be hard work to persevere and take charge over your eating and unlearn poor habits. Therefore, you need all the love and positivity you have inside to help you. You cannot change certain aspects of your personality. Instead of not accepting it, embrace the challenge and work harder to overcome it. Remember, you read that there is no challenge we encounter that we can't overcome. We are not set up for failure with the experiences we face. Choose to accept yourself the way you are and then lasting change can occur in the ways that matter.

## For Starters

 **Kosher Cleanse Elixir:** Drink upon waking (see page 97).

 **Daily Fitness Goal**: Jump into the upcoming week with a powerful lower body workout focusing on the glutes, hamstrings, and quads (youtu.be/afghBre8NlI). Don't forget to walk your 10,000 steps today!

## Breakfast

• **Berry Oatmeal**

## Snack

• ¾ **RX Bar**

## Lunch

• Collard wraps with 1 cup black beans, 2 tbsp. salsa, ½ mashed avocado, and cilantro

## Snack

• **Kale Chips**

## Dinner

• 1 cup unsweetened fennel tea, hot or iced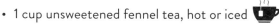
• 4 ounces Grilled Chicken
• 3 cups **Broccoli-Cauliflower Medley**
• 3 Roasted Baby Red Potatoes, seasoned with free ingredients

 **BETH'S PREP TIPS**

• Add the berries to the oatmeal as it is cooking, or add the fruit after the oatmeal is cooked.
• Defrost 1 Almond **Butter Muffin**, to eat as a snack tomorrow, and 2 **Chicken Burgers** for tomorrow's dinner.

# Day Sixteen Recipes

## BERRY OATMEAL

Yield: 1 serving

### Ingredients

½ cup old-fashioned oatmeal
¼ cup unsweetened almond milk
½ cup "tri-berries" (blueberries, raspberries, and blackberries)
1 tsp. chia seeds
1 tsp. vanilla extract

### Directions

1. Cook the oatmeal as directed in the almond milk.
2. Add the chia seeds, vanilla, and tri-berries to a bowl.

*Per serving: 220 calories, 5g fat, 0.5g saturated fat, 0mg cholesterol, 45mg sodium, 38g carbohydrates, 8g fiber, 6g protein*

## KALE CHIPS

### Ingredients

Kale, 1 head, separated into leaves and chopped
Salt and pepper, to taste
Seasonings, such as zaatar (optional)

### Directions

1. Preheat the oven to 350°F.
2. Place the kale on a baking sheet in a single layer.
3. Sprinkle with salt and pepper and any other optional seasoning, to taste.
4. Place into the oven and leave the oven door slightly ajar. Bake about 10 minutes. Keep checking on the kale chips so they do not burn.

## BROCCOLI-CAULIFLOWER MEDLEY

Yields: 6 servings

### Ingredients

1 head broccoli, washed and cut into florets
1 head cauliflower, washed and cut into florets
3 cloves garlic, minced
4 tbsp. olive oil
½ cup lemon juice
2 tbsp. dried rosemary

### Directions

1. Preheat the oven to 400°F.
2. Toss the broccoli and cauliflower with the garlic, olive oil, lemon juice, and rosemary.
3. Roast for 20 minutes.

*Per serving: 140 calories, 9g fat, 1.5g saturated fat, 0mg cholesterol, 40mg sodium, 13g carbohydrate, 4g fiber, 4g protein*

(Source: FoodNetwork.com)

# DAY SEVENTEEN

## Mindful Meditation to Start Your Day

*"Think good, and it will be good."*

—RABBI MENACHEM MENDEL OF LUBAVITCH (1789–1866)

This quote makes thinking positive thoughts sound simple, and it is. Ultimately your mindset is in your control. Allow your mind to focus on good, and good things will come. How many times can you remember when you woke up in a bad mood or had something go wrong, and it cascaded into other areas of your day? When you set a certain tone to your mood, it affects how you see things. Try to keep your thoughts positive, focus on the blessings you have, how you are present on this earth, living and breathing, along with the fact that you are doing something great for yourself each day on my diet. Ultimately, being grateful of all the good you have will breed more happy things into your life.

## For Starters

 **Kosher Cleanse Elixir:** Drink upon waking (see page 97).

 **Daily Fitness Goal:** Balance today by working out your upper body with this routine targeting your arms, shoulders, and upper back—no equipment required (youtu.be/CRGrcSDhynQ). Plus, get in your steps today!

## Breakfast

- **Lemon and Mint Cucumber Smoothie**

## Snack

- 6 ounces grass-fed plain Greek yogurt with ½ cup cubed cantaloupe

## Lunch

- **Raw Kale Salad with Sprouted Quinoa and Pumpkin Seeds**

## Snack

- 1 **Almond Butter Muffin**

## Dinner

- 1 cup unsweetened mint tea, hot or iced
- 2 **Chicken Burgers** with **Tomato Zoodles** and ¾ cup cubed roasted butternut squash

### BETH'S PREP TIPS

- Prepare the **Chia Yogurt** for breakfast tomorrow.
- Defrost ½ cup of **Lentil Soup** for dinner tomorrow.

# Day Seventeen Recipes

## LEMON AND MINT CUCUMBER SMOOTHIE

Yield: 1 serving

### Ingredients

1 cup unsweetened almond milk
¼ cup fresh lemon juice
½ avocado
5 large mint leaves
1 small banana
½ cucumber about 3 inches long

### Directions

Combine all ingredients in a blender until smooth.

*Per serving: 191 calories, 13g fat, 2g saturated fat, 167mg sodium, 0mg cholesterol, 19g carbohydrate, 6g fiber, 3g protein*

## RAW KALE SALAD WITH SPROUTED QUINOA AND PUMPKIN SEEDS

Yield: 1 serving

### Ingredients

½ bunch (about 6 cups) kale leaves, chopped and de-stemmed
Salt (optional)
¼ avocado
½ cup cooked quinoa
1 tbsp. **Toasted Tamari Pumpkin Seeds**
**Tahini Dressing**

### Directions

1. Place the kale in a large bowl and massage for about 2 minutes to help soften the leaves. A little salt can help pull out some of the kale juices and soften it up a bit as well.
2. Pransfer the kale to fresh bowl, discarding any liquid, and mix with up to 2 tbsp. **Tahini Dressing**. Toss with the quinoa and the **Toasted Tamari Pumpkin Seeds**. Top with avocado.

*Per serving: 459 calories, 14g fat, 2g saturated fat, 0mg cholesterol, 522mg sodium, 70g carbohydrate, 11g fiber, 20g protein*

## TOASTED TAMARI PUMPKIN SEEDS

Yield: 1 serving

### Ingredients

½ cup raw pumpkin seeds
1 tbsp. tamari

### Directions

1. Preheat oven to 250°F.
2. Mix the pumpkin seeds and tamari and lay the seeds flat on a baking sheet. Let sit for 15 minutes so that the seeds absorb the tamari.
3. Place baking sheet in the oven and toast in the oven for 30 to 40 minutes, or until crunchy, flipping the seeds over twice to toast evenly.

*Per serving: 153 Calories, 6g Total Fat , 1g Saturated Fat, 1,1895mg Sodium, Potassium 332mg, 0mg Cholesterol, 18g Total Carbohydrate, 5gTotal Fiber, 8g Protein*

# DAY EIGHTEEN

## Mindful Meditation to Start Your Day

*"Let all who are hungry come and eat."*

—PASSOVER HAGGADAH (THE TEXT RECITED AT THE SEDER,
THE RITUAL DINNER ON PASSOVER)

The quote for today is from the story of Passover we read in the Haggadah. There is a concept of the holiday to allow people with limited means and whoever needs food to come and enjoy the Seder and eat. As I wrote in the earlier chapters, I love food. I found that my passion for food is not only about eating it. Sometimes I can boost my mood and feelings of happiness about food when I'm preparing it for others. I discovered that cooking for food pantries or other charity outlets truly provides a sense of satisfaction without feelings of guilt. This quote reminds me not to feel if I'm missing out when I skip unhealthy food choices. Take the day to do some kindness to help boost your mood and motivation. Try volunteering at soup kitchens, provide meals for those who are sick or in need, such as a friend who has had a baby, so that you develop comforts and happiness around food without feeling an urgency to eat it. It's a win-win for your mind, body, and people in need.

## For Starters

 **Kosher Cleanse Elixir:** Drink upon waking (see page 97).

 **Daily Fitness Goal**: Take a much needed rest today for optimal muscle recovery.

## Breakfast

• **Chia Yogurt** with ½ cup of your choice of fruit

## Snack

• 2 tbsp. hummus with your choice of non-starchy veggies

## Lunch

• **Avocado Mash** on 1 slice sprouted grain bread with a large salad and your choice of dressing

## Snack

• 1 sliced pear with 1 tbsp. natural peanut butter

## Dinner

• 1 cup unsweetened fennel tea, hot or iced
• **Spaghetti Squash Lasagna** with your choice of large salad with ½ cup **Lentil Soup**

---

 **BETH'S PREP TIPS**

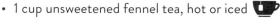

• If you didn't make the tempeh in advance, be sure you prep it today. **Marinated Tempeh** is on the menu for tomorrow's lunch!
• Take out ½ cup of **In a Jiffy Bean Salad** from the freezer for your snack tomorrow.

# Day Eighteen Recipes

## CHIA YOGURT

Yield: 1 serving

### Ingredients

1 cup unsweetened almond milk, homemade or store-bought
¼ tsp. vanilla extract
¼ tsp. ground cinnamon, optional
Added flavorings such as fruits or chocolate (optional)
¼ cup chia seeds
Berries, for serving

### Directions

1. Blend the almond milk, vanilla, and cinnamon, if desired, in a blender until smooth. Include any added flavors at this time.
2. Whisk in the chia seeds. Pour the milk-chia mixture into a jar or glass container and refrigerate at least 4 hours or overnight to let it gel. Top with berries to serve.

*Per serving (with ½ cup fruit): 310 calories, 17g fat, 1.5g saturated fat, 0mg cholesterol, 190mg sodium, 32g carbohydrates, 18g fiber, 9g protein*

## AVOCADO MASH

Yield: 1 serving

### Ingredients

½ avocado
Lemon juice, to taste
Seasonings such as cumin or red pepper flakes (optional)

### Directions

1. Mash the avocado.
2. Add a splash of lemon and any seasonings you'd like.

*Per serving: 80 calories, 7g fat, 1g saturated fat, 0mg cholesterol, 0g sodium, 4g carbohydrates, 3g fiber, 1g protein*

## SPAGHETTI SQUASH LASAGNA

Yields: 6 servings

### Ingredients

1 small spaghetti squash, sliced longwise
¾ cup part-skim ricotta cheese
¾ cup shredded part-skim mozzarella
   cheese, reserving about 1 tbsp.
¾ cup tomato sauce
1 tsp. salt
1 tsp. pepper

### Directions

1. Preheat the oven to 425°F.
2. Lay the spaghetti squash, pulp side down, on a parchment paper-lined baking sheet.
3. Roast squash for 40 minutes. When it's finished baking, spoon out the seeds, and use a fork to shred the spaghetti squash flesh into a small oven-safe dish.

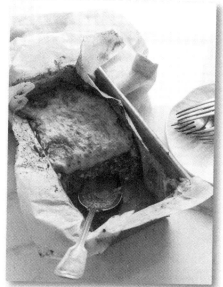

*For a color photo, see page 190.*

4. Lower the oven temperature to 350°F.
5. In a small mixing bowl, combine the ricotta, mozzarella, tomato sauce, and pepper. Stir into the spaghetti squash. Sprinkle the reserved cheese on top. Bake uncovered for about 20 to 30 minutes.

*Per serving: 118 calories, 5.6g fat, 17mg cholesterol, 243mg sodium, 10g carbohydrates, 1.8g fiber, 4.8g protein*

# DAY NINETEEN

## Mindful Meditation to Start Your Day

*"Stolen Water is Sweet, and Bread Eaten*
*in Secret is Pleasant."*
—BOOK OF PROVERBS 9:17

This quote from the *Book of Proverbs* takes us back to the concept of the evil inclination as it relates to strengthening a person's desire for unhealthy things. Think about it—once a forbidden food becomes permissible to eat, then it is suddenly not as enticing. The quote uses water, which does not have any flavor and can be boring. However, once the water was stolen and inaccessible then it became something to covet, as if it suddenly transformed into an indulgent sweet.

Don't be fooled by the tricks your mind begins to play. Foods you think you are craving are more the memories of the happy times you had while eating them. You are overthinking the urges simply because those foods are not available to you now. Remember to practice what we preached in chapter 1: think of your food craving when it pops up as nothing more than a mere thought that's fleeting—kind of like a soap bubble that will disappear as soon as you touch it.

Catch yourself when you feel you are missing out on former junk foods you loved, talk the evil inclination down and keep moving forward! *POP!*

# For Starters

 **Kosher Cleanse Elixir:** Drink upon waking (see page 97).

 **Daily Fitness Goal:** Pick your favorite HIIT workout and push your limits! Don't forget to keep walking.

# Breakfast

• Your choice of an Egg Omelet recipe from the plan with 1 cup of fruit

# Snack

• ½ cup **In a Jiffy Bean Salad**

# Lunch

• 1 serving of **Asian Tempeh Salad**

# Snack

• 1 apple with 12 raw almonds

# Dinner

• 1 cup unsweetened fennel tea, hot or iced

• 2 ounces whole wheat sourdough bread with **Rosemary Grass-fed Lamb Chops with Artichokes**

## BETH'S PREP TIPS

Prepare the Grilled Chicken for tomorrow's lunch!

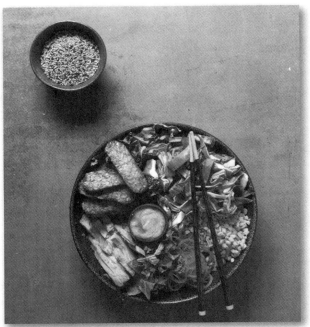

*For a color photo, see page 187.*

# Day Nineteen

## ASIAN TEMPEH SALAD

Yield: 1 serving

### Ingredients

2 to 3 cups, or more, kale
2 tsp. extra-virgin olive oil
4 slices prepared **Marinated Tempeh**
¼ cup shredded purple cabbage
½ cup farro, cooked according to package directions
2 tbsp. tuxedo (black and white) sesame seeds
2 tbsp. **Miso Dressing**

### Directions

1. Massage the kale coated in the olive oil with your hands to soften it.
2. Arrange the salad in this order: kale, tempeh, cabbage, and farro. Top with the sesame seeds and dressing.

*Per serving: 512 calories, 27g fat, 3g saturated fat, 0mg cholesterol, 353 mg sodium, 58g carbo-hydrates, 13.5g fiber, 28g protein*

## ROSEMARY GRASS-FED LAMB CHOPS WITH ARTICHOKES

Yields: 8 servings

### Ingredients

1 handful of fresh rosemary
4 garlic cloves
1 tbsp. extra-virgin olive oil
1 tsp. salt
Pinch of black pepper
1 rack of lamb (about 8 chops)
1 (6-ounce) bag of artichoke
    bottoms

### Directions

1. Preheat the oven to 350°F.
2. Place the rosemary, garlic, olive oil, salt, and pepper in a food processor and pulse to combine.
3. Rub the rosemary-garlic mixture on the lamb in a glass casserole dish.
4. Place the artichokes all around.

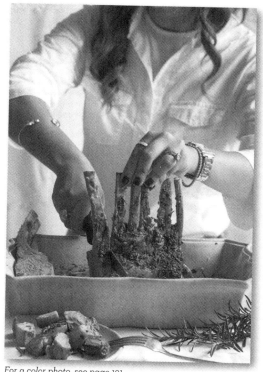

*For a color photo, see page 191.*

5. Bake, covered, about 40 minutes. Uncover and bake a few more minute to brown the chops.

*Per serving, 2 lamb chops: 150 calories, 14g fat, 2g saturated fat, 9mg cholesterol, 472mg sodium, 1g carbohydrates, 0g fiber, 3g protein*

# DAY TWENTY

## Mindful Meditation to Start Your Day

*"Act while you can:
While you have the chance,
the means, and the strength."*

—TALMUD, SHABBAT 151B

You are so close that you can taste (literally!) the success of completing the 21-day plan. Start your day with a renewed strength from seeing the finish line in your grasp. Feel the anticipation for the end and bask in the immense sense of accomplishment you are entitled to feel for your efforts. Begin to reflect on how you feel physically and emotionally. Start to relish in the benefits after following my kosher whole foods way and complete Day 20 knowing that you got this.

## For Starters

 **Kosher Cleanse Elixir:** Drink upon waking (see page 97).

 **Daily Fitness Goal:** Ease into the last day of the diet with your most empowering yoga routine, leaving you feeling proud and inspired.

## Breakfast

- ¾ cup of 1% cottage cheese with 1 cup pineapple, ground cinnamon, and 1 tsp. chia seeds

## Snack

- ¼ cup **Coconut Granola**

## Lunch

- ½ cup **Quinoa Salad** (or 2 ounces whole wheat sourdough bread)
- 4 ounces Grilled Chicken and a large salad with your choice of dressing

## Snack

- ½ cup **Roasted Chickpeas** with 2 or more Persian cucumbers

## Dinner

- 1 cup unsweetened fennel tea, hot or iced
- **Potato-Egg Salad** with **Zucchini Vegetable Soup**

### BETH'S PREP TIPS

- Use the leftover **Roasted Chickpeas** from Week 2.
- Prepare the Grilled Salmon for tomorrow's lunch, or use 100% wild salmon packed in water.

# Day Twenty Recipes

## QUINOA SALAD

Yields: 4 servings

### Ingredients

½ cup quinoa, cooked according to package directions
½ cup black beans, rinsed
1 red, orange, and yellow bell pepper, seeded and chopped
½ cup organic corn niblets
2 tbsp. chopped fresh parsley
**Cumin Dressing**

### Directions

1. In a large bowl, combine the quinoa, black beans, peppers, corn, and parsley.
2. Toss with 2 tbsp. **Cumin Dressing** per serving.

*Per serving (½ cup): 140 calories,1.5g fat, 0g saturated fat, 0mg cholesterol, 200mg sodium, 95g carbohydrates, 5g fiber, 6g protein*

## POTATO-EGG SALAD

Yield: 1 serving

### Ingredients

2 hardboiled eggs, chopped
½ cup cubed boiled potato
1 tsp. extra-virgin olive oil
Juice of ½ lemon
½ tsp. salt
¼ tsp. pepper
¼ tsp. ground cumin

### Directions

1. Combine the eggs and potatoes in a small bowl. Season with the olive oil, lemon juice, salt, pepper, and cumin.
2. Toss ingredients and serve.

*Per serving: 300 calories, 21g fat, 5g saturated fat, 515 mg cholesterol, 155 mg sodium, 9g carbo-hydrates, 18g protein*

## ZUCCHINI VEGETABLE SOUP

### Ingredients

1 tbsp. extra-virgin olive oil
1 large onion, chopped
¼ teaspoon dried thyme
¼ teaspoon dried rosemary
½ teaspoon dried basil
¼ teaspoon ground white pepper
sea salt, to taste
8 small zucchinis, halved lengthwise and sliced
6 stalks of celery, chopped
1 quart (4 cups) organic low-sodium no-chicken broth or vegetable broth
Water to add to broth as needed

### Directions

1. Heat the olive oil in a large pot over medium-high heat. Stir in the onion and cook until it's translucent. Add the thyme, rosemary, basil, white pepper, and salt.
2. Stir in the zucchini and celery, and cook until tender, about 5 minutes.
3. Pour in the broth. Bring to a boil, reduce heat, cover, and simmer 15 to 20 minutes.
4. Remove the soup from heat. Use a hand blender, or transfer in batches to a blender, and blend until mostly smooth.

*Per serving: 160 calories, 13.5g fat, 2g saturated fat, 0mg cholesterol, 560mg sodium, 16g carbohydrates, 8g fiber, 5g protein*

# DAY TWENTY-ONE

## Mindful Meditation to Start Your Day

*"Pleasant words are as a honeycomb,*
*sweet to the soul and healing to the bones."*

—BOOK OF PROVERBS 16:24

You've made it to the last day. Be sure to keep your thoughts and words pleasant. Remember that only positive thoughts will keep you moving towards what you want, weight loss and better health. Happy talk is what will allow you to feel all your accomplishments from your dieting journey. Don't belittle the tremendous impact following the plan had on your energy, mood, and health aside from fat loss. You can continue beyond the diet with the impactful diet and lifestyle habits you learned. Read further to learn how to maintain your amazing results after you complete your final day on my kosher girl's diet. Congratulations!

 **BETH'S PREP TIPS**

I advise weighing-in and taking all the other metrics to measure including, waist, hip and body fat calculations the morning of Day 22. Note them all in your Metrics Tracker and compare your results to Day 1 and Day 8.

## For Starters

 **Kosher Cleanse Elixir:** Drink upon waking (see page 97).

 **Daily Fitness Goal**: Perform a combo of everything you learned in the fitness area. Try 15 minutes of yoga, 30 minutes of HIIT, and end with 15 minutes of yoga.

## Breakfast

• **Cashew Cream Smoothie**

## Snack

• 1 apple and 12 raw almonds

## Lunch

• 4 ounces Grilled Salmon on a large salad made with ½ cup cubed beets and your choice of dressing

## Snack

• 1 **Health Warrior Chia Bar**

## Dinner

• 4 ounces **Zaatar Bronzini** with ½ cup **Wheatberry Salad** and roasted non-starchy vegetables

# Day Twenty-One Recipes

## CASHEW CREAM SMOOTHIE

Yields: 2 servings

### Ingredients

1 cup water
1 cup raw cashews
1 cup ice
1 banana
1 vanilla bean, seeds scraped (reserve the bean pod for another use),
    or 1 tsp. pure vanilla extract

### Directions

1. Pour the water over cashews and let stand until the cashews have softened, about 15 minutes. If you don't have time for this simply put the water and cashews into the blender.
2. Purée in blender on high for 3 minutes, until it's smooth.
3. Add the ice, banana, and vanilla, and blend until smooth.

*Per serving: 410 calories, 28g fat, 5g saturated fat, 0mg cholesterol, 10mg sodium, 33g carbohydrates, 4g fiber, 12g protein*

## ZAATAR BRANZINI

Yield: 1 serving

### Ingredients

1 (4-ounce) branzini fillet (or any lean whitefish fillet, except tilapia)
1 tbsp. extra-virgin olive oil
1 tsp. zaatar spice
Juice of ½ a lemon

### Directions

1. Marinate the branzini or other whitefish in the olive oil, zaatar, and lemon juice by refrigerating 60 minutes, ideally.
2. Preheat the oven to 350°F.
3. Line a baking sheet with parchment paper. Place fish fillet on the baking sheet.
4. Bake 12 minutes.

*Per serving: 230 calories, 16g fat, 2g saturated fat, 0mg cholesterol, 75mg sodium, 2g carbohydrates, 0g fiber, 21g protein*

## WHEATBERRY SALAD

Yields: 4 servings

### Ingredients

*For the Weatberries:*
½ cup wheatberries
1½ cups of water, plus more to cool
½ tsp. salt, divided

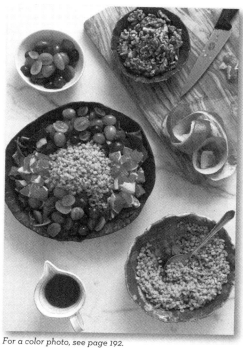

*For the Vinaigrette:*
2 tablespoons extra-virgin olive oil
1 tablespoon balsamic vinegar
Zest of half an orange
½ tbsp. fresh orange juice
¼ tsp. agave syrup
½ tsp. Dijon mustard
¼ tsp. salt
¼ tsp. curry powder
Pinch of cayenne, ground ginger,
    and black pepper

*For the Salad:*
2.5 ounces baby kale
½ cup seedless red grapes, halved
½ cup seedless green grapes, halved
1 orange, peeled, pits removed, and segmented
Salt and pepper, to taste
¼ cup raw unsalted walnuts, toasted and coarsely chopped

*For a color photo, see page 192.*

### Directions for the Wheatberries

1. Rinse the wheatberries and place them in medium pot with 1½ cups of water. Add ¼ tsp. salt.
2. Bring to a boil, then reduce to a simmer.
3. Cook, covered, about 1 hour until the wheatberries are tender.
4. Add few cups of cold water to the pot, stir, and drain.
5. Place the wheatberries in large bowl to cool.

### Directions for the Vinaigrette

1. In small jar, combine the olive oil, balsamic vinegar, orange zest, orange juice, agave syrup, Dijon mustard, ¼ tsp. salt, curry powder, cayenne, ginger, and pepper.
2. Seal tightly and shake vigorously to combine. Set aside.

*(recipe continues, page 198)*

### Directions for the Salad

1. Combine cooled wheatberries with the kale in large bowl.
2. Toss with half of the dressing, add the grapes and orange segments, and more dressing.
3. Toss again.
4. Toss in walnuts right before serving. Season with salt and pepper.

*Per serving (½ cup): 180 calories, 12g fat, 1.5g saturated fat, 0mg cholesterol, 310mg sodium, 19g carbohydrates, 4g fiber, 3g protein*

## TESTIMONIAL

An email from Andrew:

Dear Beth,

Thanks again for the three weeks cleanse, I am so happy I opted into the opportunity to try the diet. As you know, I lost twenty pounds in the weeks and to do that on a healthy cleanse that was so satisfying was an amazing feat. I felt that the advantages of the diet were that for the most part, I was surprisingly not hungry at all. It was good to learn about some new foods to eat that I would not have tried like quinoa recipes, stuff like the chia yogurt, and to use almond milk. I am doing my best to eat every three hours every day now, popping some almonds or a vegetable into my mouth. I plan on doing this cleanse again and that is the best compliment I can give.

Of course, there were some items I was not a fan of and most likely would substitute next time, like the green smoothies, but those were just minor bumps in the road. Overall, the experience was something I looked forward to each day!

*"L'fum tzara agra, according to the effort is the reward."*
—BEN HEI HEI, ETHICS OF THE FATHERS 5:26

*"This is the great equalizer. It doesn't matter where you have started on the ladder of life; it matters how many rungs you've climbed. This is the true measure of man. As President Coolidge said: Nothing in this world can take the place of persistence. Talent will not: nothing is more common than unsuccessful men with talent. Genius will not; unrewarded genius is almost a proverb. Education will not: the world is full of educated derelicts. Persistence and determination alone are omnipotent..."*
—RABBI NECHEMIA COOPERSMITH

# Part Four

# THE KOSHER PATH TOWARD MAINTENANCE

---

*"A righteous man will surely fall seven times—*
*yet will pick himself right up, once again."*
—KING SOLOMON, PROVERBS, 24:16

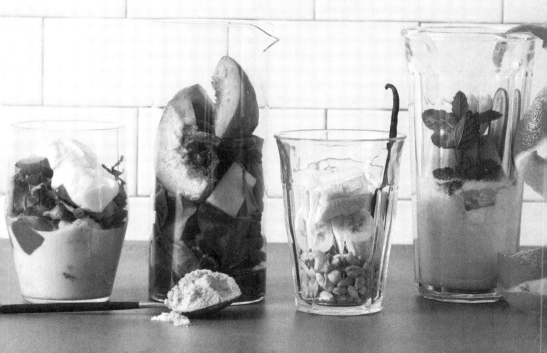

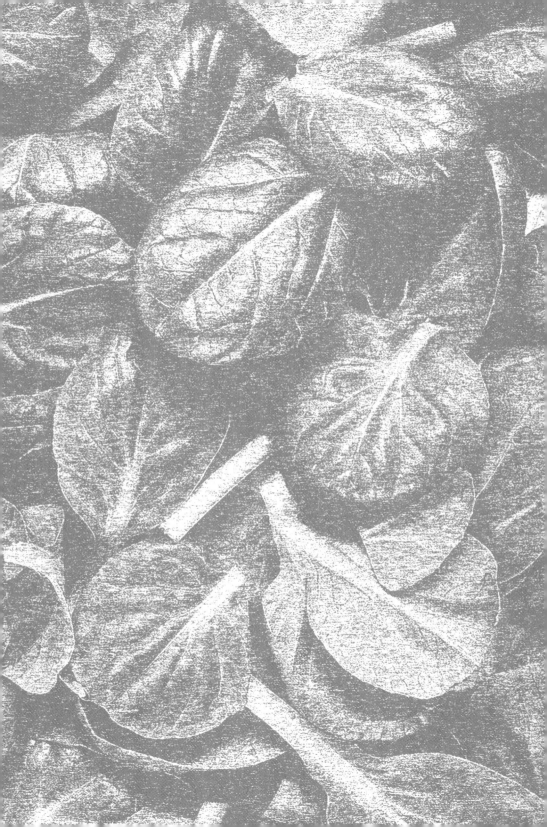

# CHAPTER SIX

# The Kosher Path
# Toward Maintenance

Life is all about the ability to get up from challenge. Greatness is
defined as getting up one more time than what you've fallen down.
The Torah defines someone who's righteous not as someone who had
succeeded, but someone who has persevered. It creates a paradigm
of what righteousness is—trying to do what's right, getting up from
failure, and keep moving forward.

—DR. YVETTE ALT MILLER

**You did it!** You reached the end of my kosher girl's diet. Following the
path of keeping clean and kosher is about the journey, not the final
destination. Hopefully, you discovered various areas of the process that
you enjoy and made you feel good. The transition into maintenance
can be more overwhelming than the feelings you had at the start of
the diet. It is understandable that as strict as you followed the meal
plan, shopped and prepped each recipe down to the last detail, and
watched the clock to be sure you ate on time during the 21 days, that
you were wondering one anxiety-provoking question: is this how I will
eat forever?

The answer falls somewhere between "yes" and "no." When you
coast through maintenance, your job is to learn your limits after
consuming foods not on the plan or as you bend rules of the diet, such
as eating any source of carbohydrate during meals or skipping one
snack per day. The goal is to listen to your mind-body cues when you

pushed too far and catch yourself at about a 2- to 4-pound gain or loss, monthly. Let's keep up those feel-good feelings along with the weight loss by following these tips for maintenance beyond the 21 days.

My Maintenance Mantra: *What You Do One Day You Simply Don't Do the Next Day*

## Redefining Your New Normal

You may not have noticed at the time, but throughout the 21 days, you created a new normal. Habits that include eating 5 to 6 times per day or opting for a clean snack such as veggies and hummus may have been impossible to fathom implementing into your life before the diet. In retrospect, you look at how successful you were in forming a new standard—the best clean and kosher monster. Confidently burst through maintenance and do not assume that you will automatically fall back to poor eating patterns and food choices. You may just as easily surprise yourself that prior cravings no longer hold the same flavor appeal.

I find it amusing when clients ask me, "Can I ever go back to eating regularly?" First, I clarify "normal." Take peanut butter, for example. I have heard how icky natural peanut butter looks when it is separated. I amend peoples' thought processes when I explain separation is healthy—the solid consistency as a result of trans fat is not normal.

Second, I rebuff with another question of my own. "Do you want to go back to how you ate before the diet?" Think all the way back to chapter 1. I proved that the memory of eating something is so powerful that you feel as if you are eating the food; however, the sensation is mostly in your mind. At the completion of the 21 days, assess how different you are now than who you were when you ate the food. Most likely when you choose to eat something highly processed it will no longer taste the same as you remember. Your palate is sensitized to enjoy healthy foods and warns you against eating something unhealthy by giving the feeling that food you are eating is too sweet. The gist of maintenance is listening to the directions your body is telling your mind. It is after you start to ignore the signals consistently that weight gain creeps up over time.

As a result, a reflection of being "normal" is to recognize that you do not need to eat as much of an unhealthy item as you did 21 days ago, if at all, to enjoy the flavor or feel less restricted. You learned the art of building awareness. During these critical moments you are faced with a choice: choose to appreciate the indulgence for what it is worth and recognize when you satisfied the craving with one bite or three, or go back to your old habits of ignoring the signals of your body telling you to stop. Remember, the biggest setbacks to maintaining weight result from choosing your mind over your body. Instead, use your body's cues to override your mind's power. You are now completely attuned to the conversation happening between your body and mind so that you can make the right choice—choose to listen.

## Fall Back on Your Outlets

Another method that is helpful in maintaining weight loss is to fall back on your newly learned outlets in times of challenge. You discovered patterns of exercise and meditations, self-affirmation, and other practices that benefit both the mind and body. These methods provide you with an external source that you can expend your anxiety or stress. A major pitfall to maintaining weight loss is emotional eating, for example. Instead of eating for reasons outside of hunger that can contribute to excess calories and weight gain, you can use your healthy lifestyle tools to refocus and reconnect in times of stress with what you learned about what to eat and how to live. If you allow it, these mind and body exercises will become your way of coping with daily pressures instead of food, paving the way for weight maintenance.

## The Recommended Breakdown During Maintenance

Although you may have used the Meal Exchange List as a reference tool if you had to make substitutions during the 21 days, it will be your go-to reference during maintenance. Here are some examples of how you can be flexible during maintenance:

▶ You can opt to make your snacks any of the food combinations and not limit to only one nut option per day, for example.

▶ You can choose to take away one snack if you are sincerely not hungry for it, as long as you do not go over four hours without eating and do not find yourself too hungry later on in the day or munching on foods more often.

▶ You can opt to have any source of portioned carbohydrate during any of the meals.

▶ You can choose to have a mindful portioned treat more than one time per week, but you would not eat it every day.

One effective motivator that helps keep you living within the overall guidelines of my diet is reading through your Wellness Planner. Consider the planner your source to flip back through at times when you need a motivational boost during maintenance to remind yourself of how good you felt while on a diet. It helps to create your list of non-negotiables or strategies that become so much a part of you that you would never think of going back. For example, you eat whole grains versus refined grains; you eat veggies as part of your meals; you use natural sweeteners or no sweeteners in your coffee; no one messes with your fitness routines, and so on. The consistency of small positive habits that you keep over time are the critical components that guide weight maintenance.

Here are some "non-negotiable suggestions" to keep your mind focused and the weight off:

▶ Work in the kosher principles of mindfulness and spirituality daily to keep centered around intuitive eating.

▶ Be accountable to yourself by continuing to write in the Wellness Planner.

▶ Stick with the food groups and nutrient combination advised for meals and snacks.

▶ Commit to a fitness routine, which is a proven way to maintain weight.

▶ Choose forms of activity that you did while following the diet or branch out and discover your fitness favorites.

The specific suggestions for maintenance are not a one-size-fits-all approach. You may find that adding more grains in snacks and meals causes you to feel bloated or your weight creeping up over four pounds at the one-month weigh-in. In that case, you simply tighten up the flexibility in certain areas you may have given yourself too much leeway. Remember: maintaining weight is about adjusting small tweaks at a few places and not typically performing a huge fix in your diet. Perhaps eating fewer grain options during the day, incorporating an additional snack, or reeling in a treat you were eating too often would be enough to get the scale to go back down. Allowing yourself a range of 2 to 4 pounds up or down is considered a realistic maintenance goal. At the next weigh-in, observe if your adjustments worked and the weight went back down. If so, you can choose to stick to the tweaks or work in other flexibilities until the next weigh in and so forth.

In other words, during the 21 days, you learned the optimal way of eating. During maintenance, you are learning your limits. You owe it to yourself to build on the principles you learned on my kosher girl's diet and honestly listen when you have had enough of a treat or if eating something does not work for you. It is about listening to the cues of your body and acting on them, rather than ignoring them and causing weight regain. If you feel you slipped beyond what a few tweaks can fix then no worries. Simply follow the complete 21 days again to get back on track.

## The Importance of Support

A typical positive feedback of my 21-day plan is the camaraderie of support on a group What's App chat I created for fellow followers. As I continued to hand out the program to other people, many connected with former kosher girl dieters for added support. I wholeheartedly encourage you to find partners, family members, and friends to support you throughout your goals to keep healthy and maintain your weight. Peer support is also proven in research to be beneficial in research for weight management.[38] Although ultimately you are your own most powerful motivator, another cheerleader is a bonus to get you through challenging times. For this reason, I established a Facebook group for the book. Feel free to join for coaching from fellow followers and the Beth Warren Nutrition team.

## LYNN'S STORY

There are always things that you can choose to carry along with you through life beyond the 21 days to keep you on track. Whether it be always incorporating vegetables at every meal, eating on a timed schedule, or rotating your carb choices, you are never without something you can do to maintain your weight. In Lynn's story, you will hear her method of maintaining her weight loss for the past three years. Aside from check-ins every three months with me, she still writes her food logs regardless of whether the option was the cleanest choice. Once she sees she is at the upper level of her maintenance weight, Lynn only buckles down on a few areas, such as increasing her minimal exercise of four days per week that slipped, including both snacks that she may have been omitting and syncing treats when she dines at restaurants more often than usual. At every subsequent weigh-in, she was always back at her optimal weight. She found the balance. And hopefully you can learn through her story how to find yours.

Lynn H., age 56

*I started with Beth Warren Nutrition in May of 2014. I was at a point in my life where I knew I needed to lose the elusive 15 to 20 pounds! I was now in my fifties, and although I considered myself a person who has always been in good shape due to a lifestyle of exercise and pretty healthy eating, I still could stand to lose 15 to 20 pounds. The blood pressure had been creeping up, and my clothes were getting pretty snug. I pretty much wore a size 4/6 most of my adult life, but now was fitting all too well into a size 8! I did not like this! So again, knowing I needed to make some changes, I made an appointment with Beth. I am not a kosher girl, nor am I Jewish, but Beth's whole food strategy and focus on intuitive eating resonated with me. From the first day I met the Beth and the girls, I knew I was on the right track. With Beth's emphasis on portion control and logging of food on a daily basis, I was on my way. I learned you have to eat to lose weight!! How great is that! Well, the weight came off fairly quickly and had stayed off for over three years. I believe my success is because I continue to log my food intake daily and that I am accountable to Beth and the team. Their continued encouragement and support has sustained me on my journey, and I am forever grateful for that!*

# EXERCISES

The following circuit training and yoga exercises will be helpful in conjunction with your Kosher diet.

# CIRCUIT TRAINING

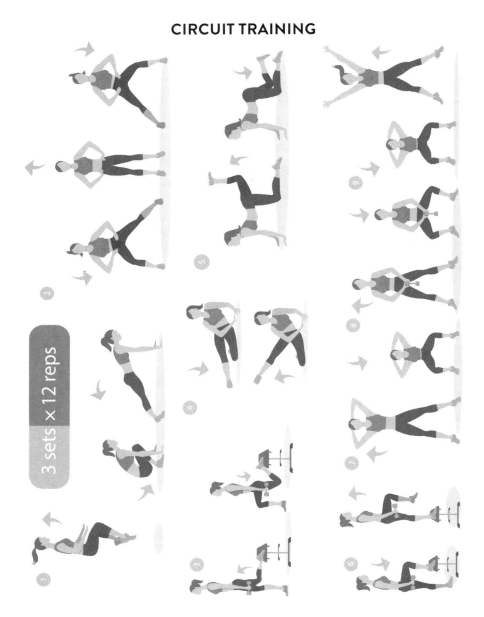

3 sets × 12 reps

# CIRCUIT TRAINING

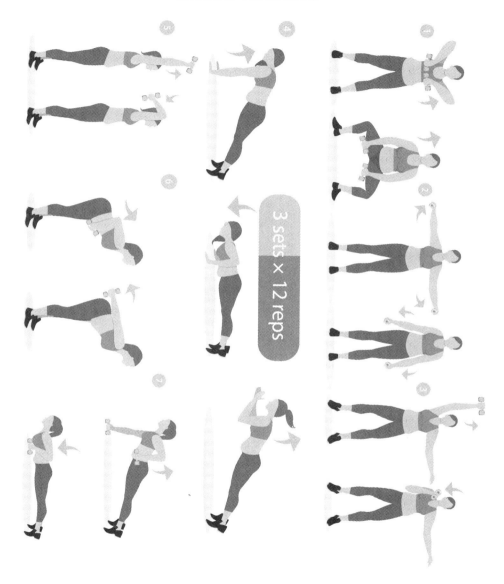

3 sets × 12 reps

## CIRCUIT TRAINING

# Lose Weight
### fast & easy

**1** 20 crunches

**2** 3 sets 8 reps

**3** 3 sets 8 reps

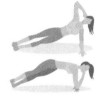

**4** 4 sets 12 reps

**5** 20 sumo squats

**6** 4 sets 12 reps

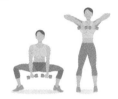

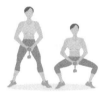

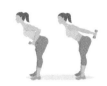

**7** 20 reverse jack-knife

**8** 3 sets 8 reps

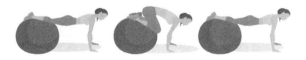

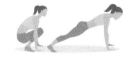

## CIRCUIT TRAINING

# Butt and Leg Workout

**1** 15 donkey kicks

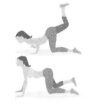

**2** 4 sets 12 reps

**3** 3 sets 8 reps

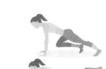

**4** 20 sumo squats

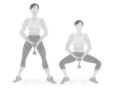

**5** 6 sets 10 reps

**6** 4 sets 10 reps

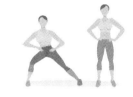

**7** 20 squat jump

**8** 5 sets 12 reps

**9** 4 sets 12 reps

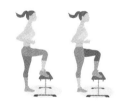

## CIRCUIT TRAINING

# Ab Crunch

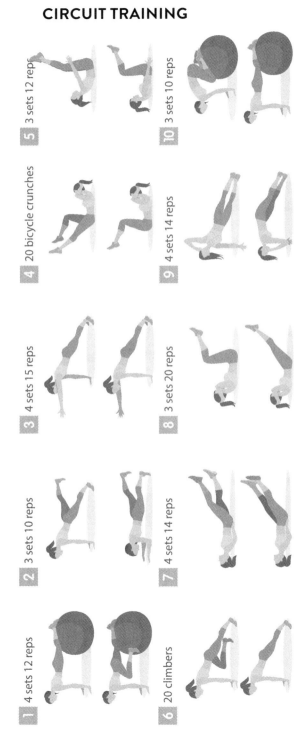

1 — 4 sets 12 reps
2 — 3 sets 10 reps
3 — 4 sets 15 reps
4 — 20 bicycle crunches
5 — 3 sets 12 reps
6 — 20 climbers
7 — 4 sets 14 reps
8 — 3 sets 20 reps
9 — 4 sets 14 reps
10 — 3 sets 10 reps

## CIRCUIT TRAINING

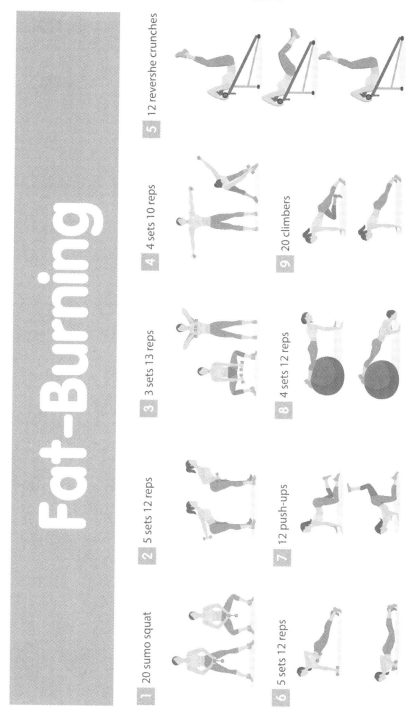

**Fat-Burning**

1 20 sumo squat

2 5 sets 12 reps

3 3 sets 13 reps

4 4 sets 10 reps

5 12 revershe crunches

6 5 sets 12 reps

7 12 push-ups

8 4 sets 12 reps

9 20 climbers

## CIRCUIT TRAINING

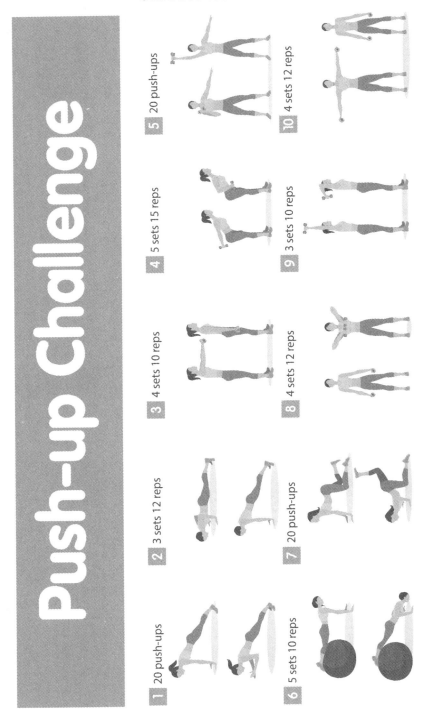

**Push-up Challenge**

1 20 push-ups

2 3 sets 12 reps

3 4 sets 10 reps

4 5 sets 15 reps

5 20 push-ups

6 5 sets 10 reps

7 20 push-ups

8 4 sets 12 reps

9 3 sets 10 reps

10 4 sets 12 reps

# YOGA

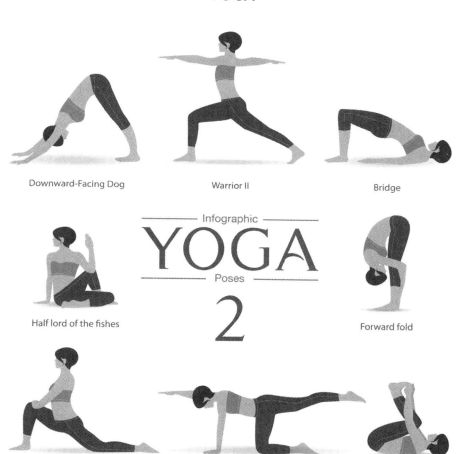

Downward-Facing Dog

Warrior II

Bridge

Half lord of the fishes

Infographic
YOGA
Poses
2

Forward fold

Low lunge

Balancing the Cat

Happy baby

# YOGA

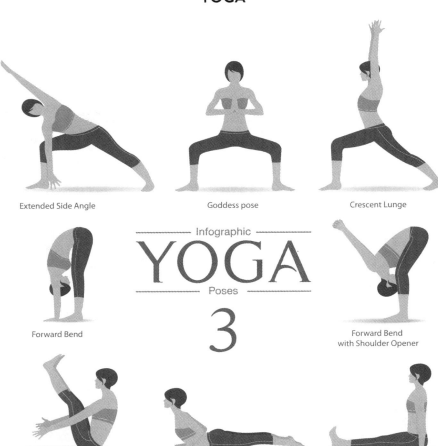

Extended Side Angle

Goddess pose

Crescent Lunge

Infographic
YOGA
Poses
3

Forward Bend

Forward Bend
with Shoulder Opener

Boat

Sun Salutation

Staff Pose

## YOGA

Awkward

Bird of paradise Revolved

Standing Knee to Chest

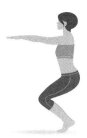

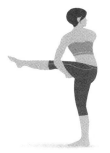

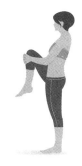

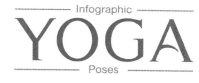

Infographic
# YOGA
Poses
## 4

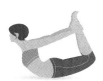

Bow

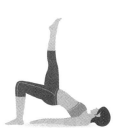

Camel

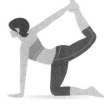

Bow Half

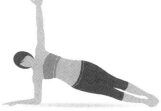

Plank Dolphin Side

Bridge Leg Up

## YOGA

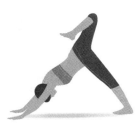

Downward Dog Leg up Stack Hips

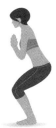

Chair Prayer

Scorpion

Chair Twist

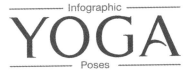

Infographic
YOGA
Poses
5

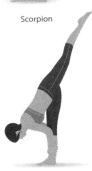

Splits Standing

Headstand Tripod Knees on Elbows

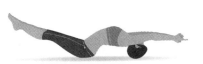

Fish

Seated Forward Bend

## YOGA

Plank Upward

Knee Pile Bind

Puppy Extended

Infographic

# YOGA

Poses

6

Shoulderstand

Standing Knee to Chest

Staff Inverted

Wild Thing

Headstand Tripod

# YOGA

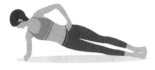

Side Plank

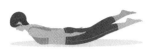

Locust Pose

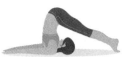

Plow

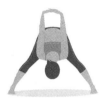

WIDE LEGGED FORWARD BEND

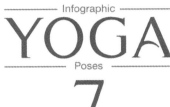

Infographic

## YOGA
Poses

7

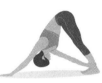

Downward Dog Twist

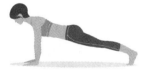

Full Plank

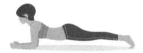

Elbow Plank

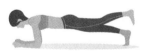

One Leg Plank

# FOODS

According to my kosher girl's diet, try to buy packaged foods that are made with whole food ingredients and kosher certified. They can be found in many standard and wholesale supermarkets like Stop and Shop, BJ's, and Costco, along with specialty markets such as Whole Foods, Trader Joe's, or online with a quick Google search, on Amazon. com and websites like jet.com.

Please keep in mind that manufacturers change their ingredients from time to time and sometimes lose kosher certification. Although I recommend these brands, get in the habit of reading food labels. Over time, products may change or companies introduce new products that are not a guaranteed fit for your weight goals.

Please keep in mind this is not an all-encompassing list. You can refer to the descriptions in this chapter and make quality whole food kosher choices on your own.

▶ ITALICS indicate ingredients that may have been left over from a purchase in a previous week.

▶ Each week requires an abundance of Non-Starchy Vegetables to make salads for meals as indicated, aside from those identified individually on the shopping list. Refer to Non-Starchy Vegetables in the Meal Exchange List for options.

▶ Some ingredient amounts are either the amount per serving to eat on the meal plan, the amount required for a recipe or the amount needed for the entire 21 days, as referenced.

Here are some ingredients to purchase that will be used throughout the 21 days for seasoning. The spices are referenced on the applicable week as well:

▶ Spices: Salt, Sea Salt, Kosher Salt, White Pepper, Black Pepper, Cumin, Chili Powder, Oregano, Onion Powder, Cinnamon, Crushed Red Pepper, Basil, Coarse Black Pepper, Hot or Sweet Paprika, Garlic Powder, Granulated Garlic, Paprika, Turmeric, Cayenne Pepper, Zaatar, Cajun Seasoning, Parsley, Curry Powder, Coriander, Thyme, Rosemary

▶ Optional After-Dinner Snack Ingredients Not Listed: Frozen Cherries, Frozen Grapes, +70% dark chocolate, Apples, Unsweetened Apple Sauce

| Section | Food | Amount | Clean and Kosher Brand Suggestions |
|---------|------|--------|-----------------------------------|
| **WEEK ONE** | | | |
| Fridge | Almond Milk, Unsweetened | 1 bottle | Califia Farms |
| Fridge | Eggs | 1 dozen | Pasture Raised |
| Fridge | Grass-Fed Plain Greek Yogurt | 18 oz. | Stonyfield 100% Grass Fed Greek Yogurt |
| Fridge | Hummus | 4 tbsp. | Hope Original Hummus |
| Fridge | Peach | 2 | |
| Fridge | Pure Tahini Paste | 1 container | Achva Organic Tahini |
| Fridge | Scallions | 2 | |
| Frozen | Frozen Cauliflower Florets | ½ cup | |
| Frozen | Frozen French Style String Beans | 1 lb. | |
| Frozen | Frozen Mango Chunks | ¼ cup | |
| Frozen | Frozen or Fresh Edamame | 1 lb. | Cascadian Farm Organic |
| Frozen | Frozen Sliced Peaches | 2 cups | |

| Section | Food | Amount | Clean and Kosher Brand Suggestions |
|---------|------|--------|-------------------------------------|
| Frozen | Peas (Frozen variety preferred) | ½ cup | |
| Fish | Branzino fillet (or any lean white fish fillet except tilapia) | 4 oz. | |
| Fish | Grilled Wild Salmon or 1 can Wild Salmon | 1 lb. + 4 oz. | |
| Meat | Brisket | 2½ lbs. | GrowandBehold.com |
| Meat | Chicken Breast | 4–6 oz. | GrowandBehold.com |
| Meat | Chopped Turkey | 1 lb. | GrowandBehold.com |
| Meat | Ground White Meat chicken | 1 lb. | GrowandBehold.com |
| Pantry | Agave or Maple Syrup | ⅔ cup | Wholesome Organic Blue Agave Syrup |
| Pantry | Almond Butter | 1 tbsp. (1 container) | Justin's Classic Almond Butter and/or Squeeze Variety; Sunbutter®, Barneys® (No Sugar or Flavor Added) |
| Pantry | Almonds, raw | 6 oz. + 1 cup | |
| Pantry | Apple Cider Vinegar | 1 bottle | Bragg's Organic Raw and Unfiltered Apple Cider Vinegar |
| Pantry | Baking Powder | 2 tsps. | |
| Pantry | Balsamic Vinegar | 1 bottle | Natural Earth Organic Balsamic Vinegar |
| Pantry | Black Beans | 3 (15-oz.) cans | Eden Foods Organic Black Beans No Salt Added |
| Pantry | *Cajun Seasoning* | 1 bottle | |
| Pantry | Cashews, raw | 6 ounces | |
| Pantry | Cashews, raw | 2 cups + 10 cashews | |
| Pantry | Cashews, raw, chopped | 1 cup | |
| Pantry | Chia Seeds | 1 tsp. + ¼ cup + 4 tbsp. | Nature's Intent |

| Section | Food | Amount | Clean and Kosher Brand Suggestions |
|---------|------|--------|------------------------------------|
| Pantry | Chickpeas | 1 (15-oz.) can | Eden Foods Organic Garbanzo Beans No Salt Added |
| Pantry | *Chili Powder* | 1 bottle | |
| Pantry | *Cinnamon* | 1 bottle | |
| Pantry | *Coarse Salt* | 1 bottle | |
| Pantry | Coconut Oil | 3 tbsp. | Spectrum Naturals Organic Coconut Oil |
| Pantry | Coconut Sugar | ⅓ cup | Health Garden Coconut Sugar |
| Pantry | *Coriander* | 1 bottle | |
| Pantry | *Crushed Red Pepper* | 1 bottle | |
| Pantry | *Cumin* | 1 bottle | |
| Pantry | Dark chocolate chips, optional | 1 bag | California Gourmet 70% dark chocolate chips |
| Pantry | Dijon Mustard | 1 bottle | Simply Balanced Organic Dijon Mustard (Target) |
| Pantry | Dried Cherries | ⅛ cup | |
| Pantry | Dried cranberries, optional | 2 cups | Made in Nature Dried Cranberries, Unsulphured |
| Pantry | Extra Virgin Olive Oil | 1 bottle | Kirkland Organic Extra Virgin Olive Oil |
| Pantry | Flax Seed, Ground | 1 container | Spectrum Organic Ground Flaxseed |
| Pantry | Grass Fed Whey Protein Powder | 2 scoops | Terra-Whey Protein Powder |
| Pantry | Health Warrior Chia Bar | 1 bar | Health Warrior Chia Bar |
| Pantry | *Himalayan Sea Salt* | 1 bottle | |
| Pantry | Honey | 1 tsp. | Wholesome Organic Honey |
| Pantry | Kidney Beans | 2 (15-oz.) cans | Eden Foods Organic Kidney Beans No Salt Added |
| Pantry | Kind Bar, Variety under 5g sugar | 1 bar | KIND |
| Pantry | *Kosher Salt* | 1 bottle | |

| Section | Food | Amount | Clean and Kosher Brand Suggestions |
|---------|------|--------|-----------------------------------|
| Pantry | Low Sodium Organic Vegetable Broth | 32 fl. oz. | Imagine |
| Pantry | Mary's Gone Crackers | 10 crackers | Mary's Gone Crackers |
| Pantry | Molasses | 1 tsp. | Plantation Blackstrap Molasses Unsulfured |
| Pantry | Nonstick Cooking Spray | 4.4 fl. oz. | Chosen Foods Avocado Oil Spray, Spectrum Olive Oil Spray |
| Pantry | *Onion Powder* | 1 bottle | |
| Pantry | *Oregano* | 1 bottle | |
| Pantry | Organic Corn Niblets | 1 (15-oz.) can | Westbrae Natural Organic Corn |
| Pantry | Organic Popcorn Kernels | 1 bag | Arrowhead Mills |
| Pantry | *Paprika* | 1 bottle | |
| Pantry | Pecans, raw | 2 cups | |
| Pantry | Pine Nuts | ½ cup | |
| Pantry | Pistachios, raw | 23 (½ oz.) | |
| Pantry | Prune Juice | 1 bottle, small | |
| Pantry | Pumpkin Seeds, raw and shelled | 1 oz. | |
| Pantry | Pure Vanilla Extract | 1 bottle | Simply Organic Pure Vanilla Extract |
| Pantry | Quinoa | 1 cup | Kirkland Organic Quinoa 4.5 lbs. |
| Pantry | Red Wine Vinegar | ⅛ cup | |
| Pantry | Red Wine, Optional | 1 bottle | |
| Pantry | Rice Vinegar | 1 bottle (12 tbsp.) | Eden Foods Brown Rice Vinegar |
| Pantry | Rolled Oats | 32 oz. | Bob's Red Mill Rolled Oats |
| Pantry | *Salt* | 1 bottle | |
| Pantry | *Sea Salt* | 1 bottle | |

| Section | Food | Amount | Clean and Kosher Brand Suggestions |
|---------|------|--------|------------------------------------|
| Pantry | Sesame oil | 8 fl. oz. | Spectrum Naturals Organic Sesame Oil |
| Pantry | Split Red Lentils | 1 cup | Arrowhead Mills Organic Red Lentils |
| Pantry | Sprouted Grain Bread | 1 package, sliced | Ezekiel |
| Pantry | Tomato Paste | 1 tbsp. | Muir Glen |
| Pantry | Tomato Sauce | ½ cup | Muir Glen |
| Pantry | Tuna, canned in water | 5 oz. | |
| Pantry | Turmeric | 1 bottle | |
| Pantry | Unsweetened Shredded Coconut, optional | 2 cups | |
| Pantry | Walnut Oil | 6 tbsp. | Spectrum Naturals Organic Walnut Oil |
| Pantry | Walnut, halves | 8 (½ oz.) | |
| Pantry | White Miso | 1 lb. | Miso Master Organic White Miso Paste |
| Pantry | White Wine (for cooking) | 1 bottle | |
| Pantry | Wild Rice | 16 oz. | Lundenberg |
| Pantry | Zaatar | 1 bottle | |
| Produce | Apples | 2 whole | |
| Produce | Apricots | 3 whole | |
| Produce | Avocado | 3 whole | |
| Produce | Baby Spinach | 2 cups | |
| Produce | Basil Leaves | 4 bunches | |
| Produce | Beefsteak Tomato | 1 large | |
| Produce | Beets | 6 whole | |
| Produce | Berries | ½ cup | |
| Produce | Blueberries | 1 container, at least 1 cup | |

| Section | Food | Amount | Clean and Kosher Brand Suggestions |
|---------|------|--------|-----------------------------------|
| Produce | Brussels Sprouts | 1 lb., frozen or fresh | |
| Produce | Carrot | 2 medium | |
| Produce | Cauliflower | 2 heads | |
| Produce | Celery | 3 + stalks | |
| Produce | Cherries | 12 whole | |
| Produce | Eggplant | 2 whole | |
| Produce | Garlic | 19 cloves | |
| Produce | Ginger, fresh | 1 whole | |
| Produce | Grapefruit | 1 medium | |
| Produce | Ground Pepper | 1 bottle | |
| Produce | Kale | 4½ cups | |
| Produce | Large Collard Green Leaves | 3 leaves | |
| Produce | Lemons | 21 whole | |
| Produce | Mango | ¼ whole | |
| Produce | Mint leaves, fresh | 2 bunches | |
| Produce | Multicolored Cherry Tomatoes | 10.5-oz. container | |
| Produce | Non-Starchy Veggies | abundant for salads | |
| Produce | Onion, white | 5 whole | |
| Produce | Orange | 1 whole | |
| Produce | Orange Pepper | 2 whole | |
| Produce | Oregano, fresh and chopped | 2 tbsp. | |
| Produce | Parsley | 2 bunches | |
| Produce | Pear | 1 whole | |
| Produce | Persian Cucumbers | 4+ whole | |
| Produce | Pomegranate | 1 whole | |
| Produce | Potato | 1 whole | |
| Produce | Red Onion | 2 whole | |
| Produce | Red Pepper | 2 whole | |

| Section | Food | Amount | Clean and Kosher Brand Suggestions |
|---------|------|--------|-----------------------------------|
| Produce | Sweet Potato | 1 whole | |
| Produce | Tomato | 4 whole | |
| Produce | Whole Wheat Sourdough Bread | 1 package, sliced and frozen individually | Bread Alone |
| Produce | Yellow Pepper | 2 whole | |
| **WEEK TWO** | | | |
| Fridge | Almond Milk, Unsweetened | 1½ cups | Califia Farms |
| Fridge | Basil | 1 bunch | |
| Fridge | Greek Yogurt, Plain | ⅓ cup | |
| Fridge | Hummus | 6 tbsp. | |
| Fridge | Lemon Juice | 2.5 tsp. | |
| Fish | Wild Salmon | 4 to 6 oz. | |
| Fish | Tuna Steak | 4 ounces | |
| Fridge | Raw Sauerkraut | 2 tbsp. | Bubbie's |
| Fridge | Tempeh | 1 (8-oz.) package | Lightlife Organic Tempeh |
| Fridge | *White Miso* | 1½ tbsp. | Miso Master |
| Fridge | Cottage Cheese | ½ cup | Organic Valley Cottage Cheese |
| Fridge | Pepper Steak, Grass-Fed | 2.5 lbs. | GrowandBehold.com |
| Fridge | Mozzarella Cheese | 1 oz. | |
| Frozen | Edamame, shelled, frozen or fresh | 1 cup | |
| Frozen | Frozen Artichoke Bottoms | 2 (14-oz.) bags | |
| Frozen | String Beans, frozen or fresh | 1 lb. | |
| Meat | Chicken Breast | 4 oz. | |
| Meat | Ground Turkey | 2.5 lbs. | |
| Pantry | *Agave Syrup* | 1 tsp. | |
| Pantry | *Almond Butter* | 1 cup | |

| Section | Food | Amount | Clean and Kosher Brand Suggestions |
|---------|------|--------|-----------------------------------|
| Pantry | Almond, sliced | ¼ cup | |
| Pantry | Almonds, Raw | 1 cup | |
| Pantry | Avocado Oil | 1½ tsp. | Chosen Foods |
| Pantry | *Baking Powder* | 1 tin | |
| Pantry | *Balsamic Vinegar* | 1 tbsp. | |
| Pantry | Black Beans | 3 (15-oz.) cans | |
| Pantry | *Black Pepper* | — | |
| Pantry | Brown Mustard Seeds | ¼ tsp. | |
| Pantry | *Chia Seeds* | 1 cup | |
| Pantry | Chickpeas, fresh | 1 (16-oz.) bag | |
| Pantry | *Chili Powder* | — | |
| Pantry | *Cinnamon* | — | |
| Pantry | *Coarse Black Pepper* | — | |
| Pantry | *Cooking Spray* | — | |
| Pantry | *Crushed Red Pepper* | — | |
| Pantry | *Cumin* | — | |
| Pantry | Dates | 1 cup | |
| Pantry | Diced Tomato | 3 (15-oz.) cans | |
| Pantry | *Dijon mustard* | 3 tbsp. | |
| Pantry | *Dried Cherries* | ⅛ cup | |
| Pantry | Eggs | 1 dozen | |
| Pantry | *Extra Virgin Olive Oil** | 1 cup | |
| Pantry | Farro | 12-ounce bag | Nature's Earthly Choice |
| Pantry | *Flaxseed, ground* | 1 tbsp. | |
| Pantry | *Garlic Powder* | 1 tsp. | |
| Pantry | Health Warrior Chia Bar | 1 bar | |
| Pantry | *Honey* | 1 tsp. | |
| Pantry | Honey, Raw | 2 tbsp. | YS Eco Bee Farms |
| Pantry | *Hot or Sweet Paprika* | — | |

| Section | Food | Amount | Clean and Kosher Brand Suggestions |
|---|---|---|---|
| Pantry | Kind Bar, Variety under 5 g sugar | 1 bar | Kind Bar |
| Pantry | *Kosher Salt* | | |
| Pantry | *Kosher Salt* | — | |
| Pantry | Mixed Nuts, Raw | 1 ounce | |
| Pantry | Montreal Steak Seasoning | Optional | |
| Pantry | No Sodium Vegetable or No-Chicken Broth | 2½ cups | |
| Pantry | Nutritional Yeast | 1 tsp. | Bragg's Nutritional Yeast |
| Pantry | Oat Flour (or 3/4 cup ground oats) | ½ cup | |
| Pantry | *Oregano* | — | |
| Pantry | Organic Corn Niblets | 1 (15-oz.) can | |
| Pantry | *Organic Popcorn Kernels* | ¼ cup | |
| Pantry | Pinenuts | ½ cup | |
| Pantry | *Quinoa* | 1½ cups | |
| Pantry | Raisins or Dried Cranberries | 1 tbsp. | |
| Pantry | Red Kidney Beans | 1 (15-oz.) can | |
| Pantry | *Red Wine, Optional* | 4 ounces | |
| Pantry | *Rolled Oats* | ⅓ cup | |
| Pantry | Rosemary | ½ tsp. | |
| Pantry | RX Bar | 1 bar | RX Bar |
| Pantry | *Salt* | — | |
| Pantry | *Sea salt* | — | |
| Pantry | Sesame Seeds, Tuxedo | 2 tbsp. | |
| Pantry | Soy Sauce, Light | ⅛ cup | |
| Pantry | Sprouted Grain Wrap | 1 wrap | Ezekiel |

| Section | Food | Amount | Clean and Kosher Brand Suggestions |
|---|---|---|---|
| Pantry | Thyme | 1 sprig | |
| Pantry | Tomato Paste | 1 tbsp. | |
| Pantry | Tomato Sauce | 2 (15-oz.) cans | |
| Pantry | Tuna, canned in water | 4 oz. | |
| Pantry | Turmeric | — | |
| Pantry | Unsweetened Shredded Coconut | Optional | |
| Pantry | Vanilla Extract | 1¼ tsp. | |
| Pantry | Whole wheat sourdough bread | 2 oz. | |
| Pantry | Wild Rice | 1 lb. bag | Lundenberg |
| Produce | Avocado | 2 whole | |
| Produce | Baby Peppers | 1 package | |
| Produce | Baby Spinach | 2 oz. | |
| Produce | Banana | 2 whole | |
| Produce | Beets | 4 whole | |
| Produce | Blueberries | 1 cup | |
| Produce | Broccoli | 1+ whole | |
| Produce | Butternut Squash | 3 lbs. (2 medium) | |
| Produce | Cantaloupe | 1 whole | |
| Produce | Carrot | 1 large | |
| Produce | Cauliflower | 1 head | |
| Produce | Celery | 3+ talks | |
| Produce | Cremini Mushrooms | 2 packages | |
| Produce | Cucumbers | 2 whole | |
| Produce | Dill | 1 bunch | |
| Produce | Fresh Parsley | 1 bunch | |
| Produce | Fresh Sage | 2 tbsp. (or ½ tsp. dried sage) | |

| Section | Food | Amount | Clean and Kosher Brand Suggestions |
|---------|------|--------|-----------------------------------|
| Produce | Fresh Thyme | ½ tsp. (or ⅛ tsp. dried thyme) | |
| Produce | Garlic Cloves | 14 | |
| Produce | Greek Yogurt, Plain | 6 oz. | |
| Produce | Green Bell Pepper | 2+ whole | |
| Produce | Green Onions | 2 whole | |
| Produce | Jalapeño Pepper | 2 whole | |
| Produce | Kale | 5 cups + | |
| Produce | Lemon | 1 whole | |
| Produce | Melon | 1 whole | |
| Produce | *Mint leaves* | 1 bunch | |
| Produce | Non-Starchy Veggies | abundant for salads | |
| Produce | Onion | 6 medium/large | |
| Produce | Peach | 1 whole | |
| Produce | Persian Cucumbers | 4+ whole | |
| Produce | Plum Tomato | ¼ whole | |
| Produce | Purple Cabbage | 1 whole | |
| Produce | Radicchio | 2 heads | |
| Produce | Red Bell Pepper | 2+ whole | |
| Produce | Red Onion | 1 whole | |
| Produce | Shallots | 6 | |
| Produce | Strawberries | 8 whole | |
| Produce | Sweet Potato | 3 medium | |
| Produce | Sweet Potato | 1 whole | |
| Produce | Tomato | 1 whole | |
| Produce | Zucchini | 5 medium | |

| Section | Food | Amount | Clean and Kosher Brand Suggestions |
|---------|------|--------|-----------------------------------|
| **WEEK THREE** | | | |
| Fish | Branzino/any lean white fish, fillet | 4 oz. | |
| Fish | Flounder, fillet | 4 (6 oz.) | |
| Fish | Wild Salmon | 4 oz. | |
| Fridge | Cottage Cheese | ¾ cup | |
| Fridge | Eggs | 5 whole | |
| Fridge | Grass-fed Greek Yogurt, plain | 6 oz. | |
| Fridge | Hummus | 2 tbsp. | |
| Fridge | Mozzarella Cheese | ¾ cup | |
| Fridge | *Tempeh* | 1 package | |
| Fridge | Ricotta Cheese | ¾ cup | Organic Valley |
| Freezer | Artichoke Bottoms | 6 oz. | |
| Meat | Chicken | 4 to 6 oz. | GrowandBehold.com |
| Meat | Chicken Breast | 4 oz. | GrowandBehold.com |
| Meat | Lamb Chops | 1 rack | GrowandBehold.com |
| Meat | White meat chicken, ground | 1 lb. | GrowandBehold.com |
| Pantry | Almond Butter | 1½ cup | Justin's Classic Almond Butter and/or Squeeze Variety |
| Pantry | Almond Flour | 4 cups | Bob's Red Mill Almond Flour |
| Pantry | Almond Milk, un-sweetened | 4¼ cups | |
| Pantry | Almonds, raw | 24 (½ oz.) | |
| Pantry | Apple Cider Vinegar | ⅓ cup | |
| Pantry | *Baking Powder* | 4 tsp. | |
| Pantry | *Balsamic Vinegar* | 1 tbsp. | |
| Pantry | *Basil, dried* | — | |
| Pantry | Beets | ½ cup | |
| Pantry | Black Beans, salt free or reduced salt | 1 (15-oz.) can | |
| Pantry | Black Peppercorns | 1¼ tsp. | |

| Section | Food | Amount | Clean and Kosher Brand Suggestions |
|---------|------|--------|-----------------------------------|
| Pantry | Brown Rice | ½ cup | Lundenberg Short Grain Brown Rice |
| Pantry | Cayenne Pepper | 1 tsp. | |
| Pantry | Chia Seeds | ½ cup | |
| Pantry | Chickpea/quinoa flour | 4 tbsp. | |
| Pantry | Chickpeas | 1 bag | |
| Pantry | Chickpeas, salt free or reduced salt | 1 can | |
| Pantry | Chocolate Chips (optional) | ½ cup | |
| Pantry | Cinnamon | 1 tsp. | |
| Pantry | Cooking Spray | — | |
| Pantry | Coriander | 1½ tbsp. | |
| Pantry | Corn Niblets, organic | ½ cup | |
| Pantry | Crushed red pepper | — | |
| Pantry | Cumin | — | |
| Pantry | Curry Powder | — | |
| Pantry | Desired seasoning for kale chips | — | |
| Pantry | Dijon Mustard | 1½ tbsp. | |
| Pantry | Dried Parsley | 2 tbsp. | |
| Pantry | Extra Virgin Olive Oil | — | |
| Pantry | Farro | ½ cup | |
| Pantry | Fennel Tea | 1 box | |
| Pantry | Garlic Powder | — | |
| Pantry | Ground White Pepper | — | |
| Pantry | Health Warrior Chia Bar | 3 bars | |
| Pantry | Himalayan rock salt | 1 tsp. | |
| Pantry | Honey, raw | 2 tbsp. | |
| Pantry | Mint leaves | 1 bunch | |
| Pantry | Old Fashioned Oats | ½ cup | |

| Section | Food | Amount | Clean and Kosher Brand Suggestions |
|---------|------|--------|-------------------------------------|
| Pantry | *Onion Powder* | — | |
| Pantry | Organic no-chicken broth or vegetable broth, low sodium | 1 quart (4 cups) | Imagine Organic |
| Pantry | *Paprika* | — | |
| Pantry | Peanut butter, natural | 1 tbsp. | Justin's Classic Peanut Butter |
| Pantry | *Pumpkin seeds, shelled* | 1 tbsp. | |
| Pantry | Quinoa | ½ cup | |
| Pantry | Red Kidney beans, salt free/reduced | 1 can | |
| Pantry | *Red Wine, Optional* | 4 oz. | |
| Pantry | Rosemary, dried | 2 tbsp. | |
| Pantry | *Rosemary, dried* | — | |
| Pantry | RX Bar | 1 bar | RX Bar |
| Pantry | Salsa | 3 tbsp. | Muir Glen |
| Pantry | Sliced Almonds | ¼ cup | |
| Pantry | Soy sauce, light | ⅛ cup | |
| Pantry | Split red lentils | 1 cup | |
| Pantry | Tamari | 1 tbsp. | San-J Organic Tamari |
| Pantry | *Thyme, dried* | — | |
| Pantry | Tomato Sauce | 1 (15-oz.) can | |
| Pantry | Tuxedo (black and white) sesame seeds | 2 tbsp. | |
| Pantry | Vanilla Bean | 1 pod | |
| Pantry | *Vanilla Extract* | 1 tsp. | |
| Pantry | Walnuts, raw | ¼ cup | |
| Pantry | Wheat Berries | ½ cup | |
| Pantry | *Whole wheat sourdough bread* | 2 oz. | |
| Pantry | *Zaatar* | — | |
| Produce | Apple | 2 whole | |

| Section | Food | Amount | Clean and Kosher Brand Suggestions |
|---------|------|--------|-----------------------------------|
| Produce | Avocado | 1½ whole | |
| Produce | Baby Red Potatoes | 4 whole | |
| Produce | Banana | 2 small | |
| Produce | Berries (raspberries, blueberries, etc.) | ½ cup | |
| Produce | Broccoli | 1 head | |
| Produce | Brussels Sprouts | 2 cups | |
| Produce | Butternut Squash | ¾ cup | |
| Produce | Cantaloupe | ½ cup | |
| Produce | Carrot | 1 mall | |
| Produce | Cauliflower | 1 head | |
| Produce | Celery | 7 talks | |
| Produce | Chickpeas, fresh/ BPA free can | 1½ cups + 1 (12-oz.) can | |
| Produce | Choice of 1 fruit | 1 | |
| Produce | Cilantro | 1 bunch | |
| Produce | Collard Wrap | 1 bunch | |
| Produce | Cucumber | 2 whole | |
| Produce | Garlic | 14 cloves | |
| Produce | Ginger, ground | ¼ tsp. | |
| Produce | Green grapes, seedless | ½ cup | |
| Produce | Kale leaves | 10+ cups | |
| Produce | Kale, baby | 2.5 oz. | |
| Produce | Lemon | 3 whole | |
| Produce | Lemon Juice, fresh | 1 cup | |
| Produce | Mozzarella Cheese | 1 cup shredded | |
| Produce | Non-Starchy Veggies | abundant for salads | |
| Produce | Onion | 1 small + 1 large | |
| Produce | Orange | 1½ whole | |

| Section | Food | Amount | Clean and Kosher Brand Suggestions |
|---|---|---|---|
| Produce | Orange Juice, fresh | 12 tbsp. | |
| Produce | Parsley, fresh | ½ cup | |
| Produce | Parsley, fresh | 2 tbsp. | |
| Produce | Pear | 1 whole | |
| Produce | Pepper, orange | 2 whole | |
| Produce | Pepper, red | 3 whole | |
| Produce | Pepper, yellow | 1 whole | |
| Produce | Persian cucumbers | 2+ whole | |
| Produce | Pineapple | 1 cup | |
| Produce | Potato | 1 whole | |
| Produce | Purple Cabbage, shredded | ¼ cup | |
| Produce | Red Grapes, seedless | ½ cup | |
| Produce | Red Onion | 1½ onion | |
| Produce | Rosemary, fresh | bunch | |
| Produce | Spaghetti Squash | 1 whole | |
| Produce | Strawberries/blue-berries | ½ cup | |
| Produce | Zucchini | 8 medium | |

# Wellness Planning

| WEEK: | | | | | | |
|---|---|---|---|---|---|---|
| **Sample Entry** | **Day 1** | **Day 2** | **Day 3** | **Day 4** | **Day 5** |
| **Sleep**<br>8 Hours<br>10:00 a.m.–<br>6:00 p.m. | **Sleep**<br>_____ Hours<br>_____:_____,<br>_____:_____ | **Sleep**<br>_____ Hours<br>_____:_____,<br>_____:_____ | **Sleep**<br>_____ Hours<br>_____:_____,<br>_____:_____ | **Sleep**<br>_____ Hours<br>_____:_____,<br>_____:_____ | **Sleep**<br>_____ Hours<br>_____:_____,<br>_____:_____ |
| **Eat**<br>B: 10 oz. berry<br>oatmeal<br>S1: ½ grapefruit,<br>10 cashews<br>L: 4 oz. salmon &<br>salad w/ ½ cup<br>beans<br>S2: 3 cucumbers &<br>¼ avocado<br>D: 2 chicken burgers<br>Brussels sprout<br>leaves w/ ½ cup<br>beets<br>Optional: Baked<br>apple | **Eat**<br>B:<br><br>S1:<br><br>L:<br><br>S2:<br><br>D:<br><br>Optional: | **Eat**<br>B:<br><br>S1:<br><br>L:<br><br>S2:<br><br>D:<br><br>Optional: | **Eat**<br>B:<br><br>S1:<br><br>L:<br><br>S2:<br><br>D:<br><br>Optional: | **Eat**<br>B:<br><br>S1:<br><br>L:<br><br>S2:<br><br>D:<br><br>Optional: | **Eat**<br>B:<br><br>S1:<br><br>L:<br><br>S2:<br><br>D:<br><br>Optional: |
| **Drink**<br>7 cups water<br>1 cup mint tea | **Drink** | **Drink** | **Drink** | **Drink** | **Drink** |

| Move It<br>10,000 steps<br>30 min<br>Type: yoga stretches | Move It<br>_____ steps<br>_____ min<br>Type: _____ | Move It<br>_____ steps<br>_____ min<br>Type: _____ | Move It<br>_____ steps<br>_____ min<br>Type: _____ | Move It<br>_____ steps<br>_____ min<br>Type: _____ | Move It<br>_____ steps<br>_____ min<br>Type: _____ |
|---|---|---|---|---|---|
| Mood | Mood | Mood | Mood | Mood | Mood |
| Notes<br>Feeling more energy and less bloated | Notes | Notes | Notes | Notes | Notes |
| Initial Weight<br>147 lbs | Initial Weight<br>_____ lbs | | | | |

# The Kosher Girl's 21-Day Diet Grid

| Day | Wake-up | Breakfast | Snack | Lunch | Snack | Dinner | After-Dinner Snack (optional) |
| --- | --- | --- | --- | --- | --- | --- | --- |
| Monday—Day 1 | 1 cup lemon water (hot or cold) and mint leaves. Squeeze juice from half a lemon into water. | Berry Oatmeal | ½ grapefruit with 10 raw cashews | 1 cup unsweetened green tea, hot or iced 1 large salad that includes any non-starchy vegetables 4 ounces grilled wild salmon (or 1 can wild salmon) + ½ cup kidney beans 2 tbsp. Lemon-Cumin Dressing | 2+ Persian cucumbers + Avocado Mash | 1 cup unsweetened fennel tea 2 Chicken Burgers Brussels Sprouts and ½ cup Beet Salad | 1 small fruit |
| Tuesday—Day 2 | 1 cup lemon water (hot or cold) and mint leaves. Squeeze juice from half a lemon into water. | Anti-Inflammatory Omelet with diced non-starchy vegetables + 1 pear | 1 small orange with 12 raw almonds | 1 cup unsweetened fennel tea, hot or iced Quinoa Salad 2 tbsp. Lemon-Cumin Dressing | 2 tbsp. hummus + 1 medium carrot | 1 cup unsweetened fennel tea, hot or iced 4 ounces Zaatar Branzini 1 Roasted Eggplant Tahini Drizzle ½ Roasted Sweet Potato | 1 cup unsweetened applesauce |
| Wednesday—Day 3 | 1 cup lemon water (hot or cold) and mint leaves. Squeeze juice from half a lemon into water. | 6 ounces plain Greek yogurt ½ cup Coconut Granola ½ cup peaches | 1 tbsp. almond butter + 2 or more celery stalks | 1 cup unsweetened fennel tea, hot or iced 4 ounces Tuna-Avocado Large green salad with ½ cup beets 2 tbsp. Miso Dressing | 1 Health Warrior Chia Bar | 1 cup unsweetened fennel tea, hot or iced 4 ounces Kale Pesto Salmon 1 cup Spicy Edamame in pods with Roasted Turmeric Cauliflower | 2 tbsp. sunflower seeds |

| Day | Wake-up | Breakfast | Snack | Lunch | Snack | Dinner | Snack | After-Dinner Snack (optional) |
|-----|---------|-----------|-------|-------|-------|--------|-------|-------------------------------|
| Thursday— Day 4 | 1 cup lemon water (hot or cold) and mint leaves. Squeeze juice from half a lemon into water. | **Kale Avocado Smoothie** | *Kind Bar* under 5g sugar variety | 1 cup unsweetened green tea, hot or iced ½ avocado (mashed with juice of ½ lemon, cumin, and red pepper flakes) 1 slice sprouted grain bread, toasted **Tomato Salad** | 2 tbsp. hummus + 2 or more cucumbers | 1 cup unsweetened fennel tea, hot or iced **Collard Wraps with Turkey Meatball, Avocado, and Dijon** 1 small baked potato with skin on | | 12 frozen grapes |
| Friday— Day 5 | 1 cup lemon water (hot or cold) and mint leaves. Squeeze juice from half a lemon into water. | 1 cup **Chia Yogurt** with ½ cup sliced strawberries/ blueberries | 12 cherries + 8 walnut halves | 2 **Gal's Black Bean Burger** on a large salad with non-starchy vegetables 2 tbsp. **Miso Dressing** | 3 tbsp. guacamole + 1 or more red, yellow, and/ or orange bell peppers | 1 cup unsweetened fennel tea, hot or iced 3 ounces **Organic Grass-fed Brisket** ½ cup **Wild Rice**, cooked (or 2 ounces challah sourdough, if mandatory) **Garlic Mustard String Beans** | | ½ ounces 70% dark chocolate |
| Saturday— Day 6 | 1 cup lemon water (hot or cold) and mint leaves. Squeeze juice from half a lemon into water. | 2 **Oat Apple Muffins** | ½ ounces pumpkin seeds (pepitas) with 3 fresh apricots | 1 cup unsweetened green tea, hot or iced 4 ounces Grilled Chicken Breast and **Fennel Salad In a Jiffy Salad** (or 2 ounces challah sourdough, if mandatory) | 2 cups **Kale Chips** with 1 tbsp. nutritional yeast | 1 cup unsweetened fennel tea, hot or iced **Spanish Omelet** 1 cup fresh organic popcorn | | 1 small fruit |

| Day | Wake-up | Breakfast | Snack | Lunch | Snack | Dinner | After-Dinner Snack (optional) |
|---|---|---|---|---|---|---|---|
| Sunday— Day 7 | 1 cup lemon water (hot or cold) and mint leaves. Squeeze juice from half a lemon into water. | ½ **Detox Protein Smoothie** with 1 cup cubed melon | ¼ mango with 23 raw pistachios | Tuna on a large salad with tons of non-starchy vegetables 10 Mary's Gone Crackers ½ cup peas (frozen, raw) 2 tbsp. **Balsamic Dressing** | 1 grass-fed 0% plain Greek yogurt with ½ cup blueberries | 1 cup unsweetened fennel tea 2 cups **Lentil Soup Turmeric Cauliflower** | 1 cup unsweetened applesauce |
| Monday— Day 8 | 1 cup lemon water (hot or cold) and mint leaves. Squeeze juice from half a lemon into water. | **Spinach and Mushroom Omelet** with 1 cup cubed melon | 100 cal. pack mixed nuts (e.g., ½ ounces of any nut combo, such as 8 walnuts, or 10 cashews, or 10 pecans) and non-starchy vegetables | 2 cup **Vegetarian Chili with Quinoa** Large salad filled with non-starchy vegetables 2 tbsp. your choice of dressing | 1 Health Warrior Chia Bar | 1 cup unsweetened fennel tea 4 ounces **Turkey Meat Sauce** and **Tomato Zoodles** 1 cup **Butternut Squash Soup** | 2 tbsp. sunflower seeds |
| Tuesday— Day 9 | 1 cup lemon water (hot or cold) and mint leaves. Squeeze juice from half a lemon into water. | **Chia Yogurt** with 1 cup of berries | 3 **Almond Date Balls** | Sprouted Grain Wrap with ½ avocado, 4 tbsp. hummus, 1 tsp. **Kale Pesto Sauce Israeli Salad** | 2 tbsp. hummus with cucumbers | 1 cup unsweetened fennel tea, hot or iced 4 ounces grilled **Honey Mustard Wild Salmon** ½ **Sweet Potato Boat** 2 cups **Lemon Artichokes** | 12 frozen grapes |

| Day | Wake-up | Breakfast | Snack | Lunch | Snack | Dinner | After-Dinner Snack (optional) |
|---|---|---|---|---|---|---|---|
| Wednes-day— Day 10 | 1 cup lemon water (hot or cold) and mint leaves. Squeeze juice from half a lemon into water. | **Overnight Oats** | ¾ *RX Bar* | 4 ounces **Grilled Tuna** on a large salad filled with non-starchy vegetables 2 tbsp. of your choice of dressing ½ cup **Butternut Squash Soup** | ¼ avocado with bell peppers | 1 cup unsweetened fennel tea 4 ounces **Turkey Burger** with a scoop of raw sauerkraut ½ cup **In a Jiffy Bean Salad** | ½ ounces 70% dark chocolate |
| Thursday— Day 11 | 1 cup lemon water (hot or cold) and mint leaves. Squeeze juice from half a lemon into water. | **3-Ingredient Pancake** | Trail Mix 100 calories, ½ ounces raw nuts and 1 tbsp. raisins or dried cranberries | **Asian Tempeh Salad** | 1 cup air-popped popcorn with 1 tsp. nutritional yeast | 1 cup unsweetened fennel tea, hot or iced 4 ounces **Miso Glazed Salmon Cauliflower Rice** roasted broccoli | 1 small fruit |
| Friday— Day 12 | 1 cup lemon water (hot or cold) and mint leaves. Squeeze juice from half a lemon into water. | **Flavorful Omelet** with 1 cup cubed honeydew | Kind Bar under 5g sugar variety | 1 cup shelled edamame Large salad filled with non-starchy vegetables ½ cup organic corn niblets 2 tbsp. **Balsamic Dressing** | ½ cup 1% cottage cheese, sprinkled with cinnamon and 1 cup of cubed cantaloupe | 1 cup unsweetened fennel tea, hot or iced 3 ounces **Pepper Steak** ½ cup **Wild Rice with Almond and Cherries** (or 2 ounces challah sourdough, if mandatory) | 1 small baked apple with cinnamon |

| Day | Wake-up | Breakfast | Snack | Lunch | Snack | Dinner | After-Dinner Snack (optional) |
|---|---|---|---|---|---|---|---|
| Saturday—Day 13 | 1 cup lemon water (hot or cold) and mint leaves. Squeeze juice from half a lemon into water. | 6 ounces plain Greek yogurt 1 cup mixed berries 1 tsp. chia seeds | ¼ avocado with cucumbers | 4 ounces Grilled Chicken **Sesame Mustard String Beans** Large salad filled with non-starchy vegetables ½ cup of beets (or 2 ounces challah sourdough, if mandatory) 2 tbsp. your choice of dressing | **3 Almond Date Balls** | 1 cup unsweetened fennel tea, hot or iced 4 ounces individual tuna Large salad filled with non-starchy vegetables ½ cup **Roasted Chickpeas** 2 tbsp. **Miso Dressing** | 2 tbsp. sunflower seeds, unsalted |
| Sunday—Day 14 | 1 cup lemon water (hot or cold) and mint leaves. Squeeze juice from half a lemon into water. | Omelet consisting of 3 egg whites plus 1 egg yolk, seasoned with your choice of spices, such as zaatar spice, and 1 peach | 1 tbsp. almond butter with 1 or more celery stalks | 2 **Gal's Black Bean Burgers** on a large salad filled with non-starchy vegetables ½ roasted sweet potato 2 tbsp. your choice of dressing | ½ cup **Roasted Chickpeas** | **Quinoa Crust Pizza** with loads of non-starchy vegetables piled on top or on the side | 1 small fruit |
| Monday—Day 15 | 1 cup lemon water (hot or cold) and mint leaves. Squeeze juice from half a lemon into water. | 2 **Almond Butter Muffins** | 18 cup mixed raw nuts with 3 large, round, no-sugar-added dried mango pieces | 2 **Baked Falafel with Tahini** on a large salad filled with non-starchy vegetables | 1 Health Warrior Chia Bar | 4 ounces **Lemon Pepper Flounder Roasted Brussel Sprouts** ½ cup cooked brown rice | ½ ounces 70% dark chocolate |

| Day | Wake-up | Breakfast | Snack | Lunch | Snack | Dinner | After-Dinner Snack (optional) |
|---|---|---|---|---|---|---|---|
| Tuesday—Day 16 | 1 cup lemon water (hot or cold) and mint leaves. Squeeze juice from half a lemon into water. | Berry Oatmeal | ¾ RX Bar | Collard Wraps with 1 cup black beans, 2 tbsp. salsa, 1/2 mashed avocado, and cilantro | Kale Chips | 4 ounces Grilled Chicken 3 cups Broccoli-Cauliflower Medley 3 roasted baby red potatoes | 1 small fruit |
| Wednesday—Day 17 | 1 cup lemon water (hot or cold) and mint leaves. Squeeze juice from half lemon into water. | Lemon and Mint Cucumber Smoothie | 6 ounces grass-fed plain Greek yogurt with 1/2 cup cubed cantaloupe | Raw Kale Salad with Sprouted Quinoa and Pumpkin Seeds | 1 Almond Butter Muffin | 1 cup unsweetened mint tea, iced or hot 2 Chicken Burgers with Tomato Zoodles 3/4 cup cubed roasted butternut squash | 1/2 cup unsweetened applesauce |
| Thursday—Day 18 | 1 cup lemon water (hot or cold) and mint leaves. Squeeze juice from half a lemon into water. | Chia Yogurt with 1/2 cup of your choice of fruit | 2 tbsp. hummus with your choice of non-starchy vegetables | Avocado Mash on 1 slice sprouted grain bread Large salad filled with non-starchy vegetables 2 tbsp. choice of dressing | 1 sliced pear with 1 tbsp. natural peanut butter | 1 cup unsweetened fennel tea, hot or iced Spaghetti Squash Lasagna with choice of large salad 1/2 cup Lentil Soup | 2 tbsp. unsalted sunflower seeds |
| Friday—Day 19 | 1 cup lemon water (hot or cold) and mint leaves. Squeeze juice from half a lemon into water. | Your choice of Egg Omelet from previous recipes with 1 fruit | 1/2 cup In a Jiffy Bean Salad | 1 serving of Asian Tempeh Salad | 1 apple with 12 raw almonds | 1 cup unsweetened fennel tea, hot or iced 2 ounces whole wheat sourdough bread Rosemary Grass-fed Lamb Chops with Artichokes | 1 small fruit |

| Day | Wake-up | Breakfast | Snack | Lunch | Snack | Dinner | After-Dinner Snack (optional) |
|---|---|---|---|---|---|---|---|
| Saturday— Day 20 | 1 cup lemon water (hot or cold) and mint leaves. Squeeze juice from half a lemon into water. | ¾ cup 1% cottage cheese with 1 cup pineapple, ground cinnamon, and 1 tsp. chia seeds | ¼ cup **Coconut Granola** | ½ cup **Quinoa Salad** (or 2 ounces whole wheat sourdough bread) 4 ounces Grilled Chicken large salad with your choice of dressing | ½ cup **Roasted Chickpeas** with 2 or more Persian cucumbers | 1 cup unsweetened fennel tea, hot or iced **Potato-Egg Salad Zucchini (Vegetable) Soup** | ½ ounce 70% dark chocolate |
| Sunday— Day 21 | 1 cup lemon water (hot or cold) and mint leaves. Squeeze juice from half a lemon into water. | **Cashew Cream Smoothie** | 1 apple with 12 raw almonds | 4 ounces Grilled Salmon Large salad filled with non-starchy vegetables ½ cup cubed beets 2 tbsp. your choice of dressing | 1 Health Warrior Chia Bar | 1 cup unsweetened fennel tea, hot or iced 4 ounces **Zaatar Bronzini** ½ cup **Wheatberry Salad** roasted non-starchy vegetables | 1 small fruit |

# Kosher Girl's Diet Calorie Goal

## Daily Caloric Requirements

| | | Calories per Day | 1,000 | 1,300 | 1,600 | 1,800 | 2,000 |
|---|---|---|---|---|---|---|---|
| | | Servings per Day | | | | | |
| Protein | 1 serving = 4–6 oz. | | 3 | 3 | 4 | 4 | 4 |
| Carbo-hydrates | Legumes | | 1 | 1 | 2 | 2 | 2 |
| | Starchy Vegetables | | 1 | 1 | 1 | 1 | 2 |
| | Grains | | 1 | 1 | 1 | 1 | 1 |
| | Oils & Fats | | 3 | 4 | 4 | 6 | 6 |
| | Non-starchy Veg | | Min 5 | Min 5 | Min 5 | Min 5 | Min 5 |
| Snacks | Nuts & Seeds[1] | | 1 | 1 | 1 | 1 | 2 |
| | Fruits[2] | | 2 | 2 | 2 | 3 | 3 |
| | Non-nut Protein | | 1 | 1 | 1 | 1 | 1 |
| | Optional Supplements[3] | Per serving suggestion/individual tolerance | | | | | |

[1] In the form of one snack "protein," refer to snack list portions
[2] As part of your snacks as "fiber," refer to snack list portions
[3] Probiotics, Vitamin D, Multivitamin, Omega-3 (EPA/DHA).
If Needed: Digestive Enzymes, Other Supplements: e.g. Collagen Powder

*Refer to Meal List for portions for Male vs. Female*

## Food Modifications

*Fruits:* You can use fruit as a carb in a meal if needed. Refer to meal list portion size.

*Fewer nuts or seeds:*
1. Eliminate nuts and seeds
2. Increase legumes by 1 serving
3. Increase protein by 1 serving

## Calculating Calorie Requirements

### BMR Harris-Benedict Formula

*Women:* BMR = 655 + (4.35 × weight in pounds) + (4.7 × height in inches), (4.7 × age in years)

*Men:* BMR = 66 + (6.23 × weight in pounds) + (12.7 × height in inches), (6.8 × age in years)

| BMR | |
|---|---|
| | × |
| Activity Factor Adjustment | |
| | = |
| Activity Adjusted Subtotal | |
| | - |
| Weight Loss Adjustment | |
| | = |
| Calorie Goal for Diet | |

### Activity Factor Adjustments

- **Sedentary Behavior or Minimal Activity** = BMR × 1.0: minimal physical activity
- **Mild Daily Activity** = BMR × 1.1: exercising less than 30 minutes, 5 times per week
- **Moderate Daily Activity** = BMR × 1.3: exercising 30-60 minutes, 5 times per week
- **Strenuous Daily Activity** = BMR × 1.5: exercising more than 60 minutes, 5 times per week

## Calorie Adjustments for Weight Loss Based on BMI

*Men*

| Maintain Weight (BMI 19-25) | BMR x Activity Adjustment |
|---|---|
| Lose Weight (BMI 25-30) | Subtract 500 calories from adjusted activity |
| Lose Weight (BMI 30+) | Subtract 500-700 calories from adjusted activity |

*Women*

| Maintain Weight (BMI 19-25) | BMR x Activity Adjustment |
|---|---|
| Lose Weight (BMI 25-30) | Subtract 300 calories from adjusted activity |
| Lose Weight (BMI 30+) | Subtract 500 calories from adjusted activity |

* Adjusted daily calorie intake: No lower than 1200–1300 unless clinical condition, body type, and BMR indicate.

# Eating Clean While Eating Out

1. **Keep up with your clean eating plan.** There is no reason to ditch your clean eating goals at the door as soon as you walk into the restaurant. Gear up with confidence that you can make the best choices for your health goals. Do not assume that you will succumb to unhealthy options. There is always an option that you can eat or modify, so be prepared to make the right ones.

2. **Browse the menu in advance.** These days it is easy to find a menu online. Check out the options so you are prepared to choose. Remember, an appetizer and a soup or salad make a great meal—just double-check that seemingly healthy items, such as "salads" include only clean ingredients (e.g., no "glazed nuts").

3. **Request to put dressings and sauces on the side.** If you are not sure what's inside a sauce, simply get it ordered on the side. If you need to add it to the dish, stick a fork inside, and drizzle onto the plate; do not dip the actual food inside or pour on top.

4. **Create your option.** Simply create your entree so that you keep your food choices balanced and clean. Feel free to ask for substitutions as you need or combine items to make a complete meal such as an appetizer and a salad.

5. **Drink water.** It may seem obvious, but it is best to drink water or unflavored seltzer as your source of fluid. Also, you can try to keep drinking before you pick up another bite or one that is less healthy. Sometimes hydrating yourself can keep you from needing to eat. You can also order hot teas, hold onto the cup with both hands, and savor the beverage to avoid overeating.

# Resources for Fitness

## Ideas for Fitness

Listed below are ideas for fitness along with the number of calories you could expect to burn in one half-hour (30 minutes) engaged in each activity. This list is provided for ideas of fun routines that may work for you. Performing an activity for half the amount of time (15 minutes) will only burn half of the calories listed. Likewise, exercising twice as long (1 hour) will yield twice as many calories burned. All are approved during maintenance; however, for the purpose of the 21-day plan, be sure your activity option is limited to low impact options or half the amount of time for high impact options. You can also use the ideas for the high impact options within the HIIT regiments (short bursts of activity) discussed in chapter 2.

## Activity

- ▶ 30 minutes, bicycling, BMX, 267
- ▶ Bicycling, mountain, general, 267
- ▶ Bicycling, leisure, 9.4 mph, 182
- ▶ Bicycling, 14–15.9 mph, racing or leisure, fast, vigorous effort, 315
- ▶ Elliptical trainer, moderate effort, 157
- ▶ Health club exercise, conditioning classes, 245
- ▶ Stretching, mild,72
- ▶ Yoga, Hatha, 79
- ▶ Yoga, Power, 126

- ▶ Ballet, modern, or jazz, general, rehearsal or class, 157
- ▶ Aerobic, low impact, 157
- ▶ Aerobic, high impact, 230
- ▶ Vacuuming, general, moderate effort, 104
- ▶ Walk/run, playing with animals, moderate effort, only active periods, 126
- ▶ Shoveling snow, by hand, moderate effort, 167
- ▶ Playing musical instruments, general, 63
- ▶ Jog/walk combination (jogging component of less than 10 minutes) (Taylor Code 180), 189
- ▶ Jogging, general, 220
- ▶ Running, 4 mph (13 min/mile), 189
- ▶ Running, 5 mph (12 min/mile), 261
- ▶ Running, 6 mph (10 min/mile), 308
- ▶ Running, 6.7 mph (9 min/mile), 330
- ▶ Running, 7.5 mph (8 min/mile), 362
- ▶ Running, 8.6 mph (7 min/mile), 387
- ▶ Running, 10 mph (6 min/mile), 456
- ▶ Running, 12 mph (5 min/mile), 598
- ▶ Running, cross country, 283
- ▶ Running, stairs, up, 472
- ▶ Basketball, non-game, general (Taylor Code 480), 189
- ▶ Basketball, general, 204
- ▶ Basketball, shooting baskets, 142
- ▶ Bowling, indoor, bowling alley, 120
- ▶ Golf, general, 151
- ▶ Golf, walking, carrying clubs, 135
- ▶ Hockey, ice, general, 252
- ▶ Martial arts, different types, slower pace, novice performers, practice, 167

- Rope jumping, slow pace, < 100 skips/min, 2 foot skip, rhythm bounce, 277 *(Advise using a jump rope within the HIIT training regimens)*
- Soccer, casual, general (Taylor Code 540), 220
- Softball, practice, 126
- Tennis, general, 230
- Volleyball, non-competitive, 6- or 9-member team, general, 94
- Walking for transportation, 2.8-3.2 mph, level, moderate pace, firm surface, 110
- Backpacking, hiking or organized walking with a daypack, 245
- Walking, household, 63
- Walking, 3.5 mph, level, brisk, firm surface, walking for exercise, 135
- Kayaking, moderate effort, 157
- Swimming laps, freestyle, fast, vigorous effort, 308
- Swimming, leisurely, not lap swimming, general, 189
- Skiing, cross country, 4.0–4.9 mph, moderate speed and effort, general, 283
- Skiing, downhill, alpine or snowboarding, moderate effort, general, active time only, 167

## Resources for Fitness Links

Here is a compilation of the resource links for fitness referenced throughout the 21 days:

- 50-minute yoga workout with Sara Stiles and Deepak Chopra youtu.be/IwprTau7-go
- Yoga weight loss and Balance workout with Sara Stiles youtu.be/uUVZAMbGtDg
- Yoga for abs and arm workout with Caitlin Turner youtu.be/7y-GvJyickA
- 45 min HIIT training and total body toning workout youtu.be/Vy9WKyN1rig

▶ Yoga for core strength with Denise Austin (requires stability ball)
youtu.be/WW2xhVF30sc

▶ Total body stretching and flexibility workout with Denise Austin
youtu.be/1nKrxZ3rk6w

▶ HIIT workout for abs and obliques
youtu.be/hyFIKDLmYyo

▶ Upper body workout (arms, shoulders, upper back). No equipment
required
youtu.be/CRGrcSDhynQ

▶ Lower body workout (focuses glutes, hamstrings and quads)
youtu.be/afghBre8NlI

▶ 30-Minute Abs & Booty-Toning Workout | Class FitSugar
youtube.com/watch?v=_ZqtZSuh5Rk

▶ 45-Minute Cardio Pilates and Strength-Training Workout | Class
FitSugar
youtube.com/watch?v=P921J1Fjoug

▶ TABATA Workout for Fat Burning & Toning / HIIT Workout No
Equipment
youtube.com/watch?v=nKlU42Z51tU

▶ Refresh, Relax, and Restore: Stretching, Pilates, Yoga Workout for
Tight Muscles
youtube.com/watch?v=Pp8UNgkcAYs

▶ 15 min "Furious Far Burner 2" Home HIIT Cardio Workout /
Burn Fat Fast
youtube.com/watch?v=jr6DuNMTQBc

▶ Fitness Blender YouTube Channel, General resource to search for
various exercise regiments
youtube.com/watch?v=jr6DuNMTQBc

| Day | Date | Time | Weight | Waist | Hip | Waist to Hip Ratio | Fat % | BMA | Notes |
|-----|------|------|--------|-------|-----|--------------------|-------|-----|-------|
| Sample Day 1 | 5/14/18 | 8:30 a.m. | 147 lbs. | 35 | 42 | .83 | 40 | 29 | I wore a black sweater and leggings, no shoes |
| Day 1 | | | | | | | | | |
| Day 8 | | | | | | | | | |
| Day 21 | | | | | | | | | |

**Metrics Tracker**

# Endnotes

1 Miller DYA. Inspiring Jewish Quotes for Rosh Hashanah. Internet: aish.com/sp/pg/Inspiring-Jewish-Quotes-for-Rosh-Hashanah.html?mobile=yes%20August%2026,%202017 (accessed August, 26 2017).

2 Wellness B. Are These Claims Kosher. Internet: berkeleywellness.com/healthy-eating/food-safety/article/are-these-claims-kosher (accessed January, 14 2017).

3 Mantzios M, Wilson JC. Mindfulness, Eating Behaviours, and Obesity: A Review and Reflection on Current Findings. Curr Obes Rep 2015;4:141-6.
Mochizuki K, Hariya N, Miyauchi R, Misaki Y, Ichikawa Y, Goda T. Self-reported faster eating associated with higher ALT activity in middle-aged, apparently healthy Japanese women. Nutrition 2014;30:69-74.
Leong SL, Gray A, Horwath CC. Speed of eating and 3-year BMI change: a nationwide prospective study of mid-age women. Public Health Nutr 2016;19:463-9.

4 Sattarshetty K. The Effect of a 'Mental Stillness' Meditation Intervention on the Mental health Risk of Primary School Aged Children. Internet: ses.library.usyd.edu.au/handle/2123/16427 (accessed March, 30 2016).
Oken BS. A Systems Approach to Stress and Resilience in Humans: Mindfulness Meditation, Aging, and Cognitive Function. Internet: pdxscholar.library.pdx.edu/open_access_etds/27002016).

5 Chabad. Basic Blessings on Food Guide. Internet: chabad.org/library/article_cdo/aid/278538/jewish/Basic-Blessings-on-Food-Guide.htm

6 Papies EK. Tempting food words activate eating simulations. Front Psychol 2013;4:838.

7 Robb-Nicholson MD, Celeste. Mindful Eating May Help With Weight Loss. Internet: health.harvard.edu/healthbeat/mindful-eating-may-help-with-weight-loss (accessed August, 11 2017).

8 Rosner F. Medicine in the Mishneh Torah of Maimonides. Jason Anderson, 1997.

9 Pedersen BK, Saltin B. Exercise as medicine, evidence for prescribing exercise as therapy in 26 different chronic diseases. Scand J Med Sci Sports 2015;25 Suppl 3:1-72.
Kirk-Sanchez NJ, McGough EL. Physical exercise and cognitive performance in the elderly: current perspectives. Clin Interv Aging 2014;9:51-62.
Denham J, O'Brien BJ, Charchar FJ. Telomere Length Maintenance and Cardio-Metabolic Disease Prevention Through Exercise Training. Sports Med 2016;46:1213-37.

10   Toledo FG, Goodpaster BH. The role of weight loss and exercise in correcting skeletal muscle mitochondrial abnormalities in obesity, diabetes and aging. Mol Cell Endocrinol 2013;379:30-4.

Caudwell P, Gibbons C, Finlayson G, Naslund E, Blundell J. Exercise and weight loss: no sex differences in body weight response to exercise. Exerc Sport Sci Rev 2014;42:92-101.

11   Rosner F. Moses maimonides: biographic outlines. Rambam Maimonides Med J 2010;1:e0002.

12   Ibid.

13   Hallsworth K, Thoma C, Hollingsworth KG, Cassidy S, Anstee QM, Day CP, Trenell MI. Modified high-intensity interval training reduces liver fat and improves cardiac function in non-alcoholic fatty liver disease: a randomized controlled trial. Clin Sci (Lond) 2015;129:1097-105.

Hazell TJ, Hamilton CD, Olver TD, Lemon PW. Running sprint interval training induces fat loss in women. Appl Physiol Nutr Metab 2014;39:944-50.

Almenning I, Rieber-Mohn A, Lundgren KM, Shetelig Lovvik T, Garnaes KK, Moholdt T. Effects of High Intensity Interval Training and Strength Training on Metabolic, Cardiovascular and Hormonal Outcomes in Women with Polycystic Ovary Syndrome: A Pilot Study. PLoS One 2015;10:e0138793.

14   Ibid.

Wewege M, van den Berg R, Ward RE, Keech A. The effects of high-intensity interval training vs. moderate-intensity continuous training on body composition in overweight and obese adults: a systematic review and meta-analysis. Obes Rev 2017;18:635-46.

Trapp EG, Chisholm DJ, Freund J, Boutcher SH. The effects of high-intensity intermittent exercise training on fat loss and fasting insulin levels of young women. Int J Obes (Lond) 2008;32:684-91.

15   Huth PJ, DiRienzo DB, Miller GD. Major scientific advances with dairy foods in nutrition and health. J Dairy Sci 2006;89:1207-21.

16   Gunther CW, Legowski PA, Lyle RM, McCabe GP, Eagan MS, Peacock M, Teegarden D. Dairy products do not lead to alterations in body weight or fat mass in young women in a 1-y intervention. Am J Clin Nutr 2005;81:751-6.

17   McAfee AJ, McSorley EM, Cuskelly GJ, Moss BW, Wallace JM, Bonham MP, Fearon AM. Red meat consumption: an overview of the risks and benefits. Meat Sci 2010;84:1-13.

18   Pimpin L, Wu JH, Haskelberg H, Del Gobbo L, Mozaffarian D. Is Butter Back? A Systematic Review and Meta-Analysis of Butter Consumption and Risk of Cardiovascular Disease, Diabetes, and Total Mortality. PLoS One 2016;11:e0158118.

19   Ibid.

20   Anonymous 2013 Partial List of Acceptable Kosher Symbols, Courtesy of Oregon Kosher. Internet: oregonkosher.org/uploads/2/1/6/3/21638982/1151183.jpg?13824167242013).

21 Garaulet M, Gomez-Abellan P, Alburquerque-Bejar JJ, Lee YC, Ordovas JM, Scheer FA. Timing of food intake predicts weight loss effectiveness. Int J Obes (Lond) 2013;37:604-11.

22 Mattson MP, Allison DB, Fontana L, Harvie M, Longo VD, Malaisse WJ, Mosley M, Notterpek L, Ravussin E, Scheer FA, et al. Meal frequency and timing in health and disease. Proc Natl Acad Sci U S A 2014;111:16647-53.

23 Martinez SM, Tschann JM, Butte NF, Gregorich SE, Penilla C, Flores E, Greenspan LC, Pasch LA, Deardorff J. Short Sleep Duration Is Associated With Eating More Carbohydrates and Less Dietary Fat in Mexican American Children. Sleep 2017;40:10.1093/sleep/zsw057.
Cardena-Villarreal VM. Relationship Between Sleep, Hunger, Cravings for Food, Sedentary Lifestyle and Weight in Adolescents. 2013

24 Brigham and Women's Hospital. Division of Sleep and Circadian Disorders. Internet: brighamandwomens.org/Departments_and_Services/medicine/services/sleepmedicine/default.aspx

25 Watanabe Y, Saito I, Henmi I, Yoshimura K, Maruyama K, Yamauchi K, Matsuo T, Kato T, Tanigawa T, Kishida T, et al. Skipping Breakfast is Correlated with Obesity. J Rural Med 2014;9:51-8.
Lowden A, Moreno C, Holmback U, Lennernas M, Tucker P. Eating and shift work, effects on habits, metabolism and performance. Scand J Work Environ Health 2010;36:150-62.
Jakubowicz D, Barnea M, Wainstein J, Froy O. High caloric intake at breakfast vs. dinner differentially influences weight loss of overweight and obese women. Obesity (Silver Spring) 2013;21:2504-12.

26 Amankwaah AF, Sayer RD, Wright AJ, Chen N, McCrory MA, Campbell WW. Effects of Higher Dietary Protein and Fiber Intakes at Breakfast on Postprandial Glucose, Insulin, and 24-h Interstitial Glucose in Overweight Adults. Nutrients 2017;9:10.3390/nu9040352.

27 Tay J, Luscombe-Marsh ND, Thompson CH, Noakes M, Buckley JD, Wittert GA, Yancy WS,Jr, Brinkworth GD. Comparison of low- and high-carbohydrate diets for type 2 diabetes management: a randomized trial. Am J Clin Nutr 2015;102:780-90.

28 Mollard RC, Luhovyy BL, Smith C, Anderson GH. Acute effects of pea protein and hull fibre alone and combined on blood glucose, appetite, and food intake in healthy young men—a randomized crossover trial. Appl Physiol Nutr Metab 2014;39:1360-5.

29 Cowen LE, Hodak SP, Verbalis JG. Age-associated abnormalities of water homeostasis. Endocrinol Metab Clin North Am 2013;42:349-70.

30 Digital Torah. Talmud, Yoma 67a. Internet: dtorah.com/otzar/shas_soncino.php?ms=Yoma&df=67a%206-30-17 (accessed June, 30 2017).

31 Pan MH, Tung YC, Yang G, Li S, Ho CT. Molecular mechanisms of the anti-obesity effect of bioactive compounds in tea and coffee. Food Funct 2016;7:4481-91.

32  Eckstein L, Adams K. Pocket Resource for Nutrition Assessment. Internet: eatright-store.org/product/59D604A4-79B0-4A2B-8548-8715860342A02013).

Institute of Medicine. Dietary Reference Intakes for Water, Potassium, Sodium, Chloride, and Sulfate. 2005.

Mahan KL, Raymond J, Raymond J, Escott-Stump S. 2011.

33  Harris A, Ursin H, Murison R, Eriksen HR. Coffee, stress and cortisol in nursing staff. Psychoneuroendocrinology 2007;32:322-30.

Chao AM, Jastreboff AM, White MA, Grilo CM, Sinha R. Stress, cortisol, and other appetite-related hormones: Prospective prediction of 6-month changes in food cravings and weight. Obesity (Silver Spring) 2017;25:713-20.

34  Sonoda JI, Ikeda R, Baba Y, Narumi K, Kawachi A, Tomishige E, Nishihara K, Takeda Y, Yamada K, Sato K, et al. Green tea catechin, epigallocatechin-3-gallate, attenu-ates the cell viability of human non-small-cell lung cancer A549 cells via reducing Bcl-xL expression. Exp Ther Med 2014;8:59-63.

35  Dietz C, Dekker M. Effect of Green Tea Phytochemicals on Mood and Cognition. Curr Pharm Des 2017;23:2876-905.

36  Boschmann M, Steiniger J, Hille U, Tank J, Adams F, Sharma AM, Klaus S, Luft FC, Jordan J. Water-induced thermogenesis. J Clin Endocrinol Metab 2003;88:6015-9.

37  Arnaoutis G, Kavouras SA, Angelopoulou A, Skoulariki C, Bismpikou S, Mourtakos S, Sidossis LS. Fluid Balance During Training in Elite Young Athletes of Different Sports. J Strength Cond Res 2015;29:3447-52.

Hackney. Improvement of Human Performance in Sport and Exercise: Nutritional Factors, Carbohydrates and Liquids. 2008;

Gandy J. Water intake: validity of population assessment and recommendations. Eur J Nutr 2015;54 Suppl 2:11-6.

38  Kulik NL, Fisher EB, Ward DS, Ennett ST, Bowling JM, Tate DF. Peer support enhanced social support in adolescent females during weight loss. Am J Health Behav 2014;38:789-800.

Verheijden MW, Bakx JC, van Weel C, Koelen MA, van Staveren WA. Role of social support in lifestyle-focused weight management interventions. Eur J Clin Nutr 2005;59 Suppl 1:S179-86.

39  Anonymous What Does Kosher Mean? Internet: koshercertification.org.uk/whatdoe .html (accessed June, 11 2017).

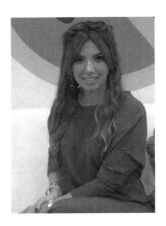

# About the Author

Nationally recognized registered dietitian-nutritionist Beth Warren—the Kosher Girl—is the founder and chief executive officer of Beth Warren Nutrition, LLC, a New York-based private practice. Beth has been sharing her kosher expertise and practical approach to healthy living for years. She has been featured on national and local television and radio programs, including Fox5, NBC's *Daytime*, and Sirius/XM Doctor's radio station, along with print and online publications, including *The NY Post*, *Women's Health*, *Glamour*, *Shape*, *Prevention*, *Men's Fitness*, and WebMD. She created a YouTube channel, Beth Warren Nutrition, and currently writes a blog featuring kosher recipes, food photos, commentary on nutrition topics in the news, and other wellness topics.